HELP NATURE TO
HEAL YOU
FROM CANCER

HELP NATURE TO HEAL YOU FROM CANCER

◆

A GUIDE ON CANCER PREVENTION, AND NATURAL AND ALTERNATIVE THERAPIES

Danuta Ryduchowski, Ph.D.

iUniverse, Inc.
New York Lincoln Shanghai

HELP NATURE TO HEAL YOU FROM CANCER
A GUIDE ON CANCER PREVENTION, AND NATURAL AND ALTERNATIVE THERAPIES

iUniverse books may be ordered through booksellers or by contacting:

iUniverse
2021 Pine Lake Road, Suite 100
Lincoln, NE 68512
www.iuniverse.com
1-800-Authors (1-800-288-4677)

ISBN-13: 978-0-595-38705-2 (pbk)
ISBN-13: 978-0-595-83087-9 (ebk)
ISBN-10: 0-595-38705-5 (pbk)
ISBN-10: 0-595-83087-0 (ebk)

Printed in the United States of America

To Casimir and Halinka

Contents

A Basic Review of the Alternative/Holistic Cancer Therapies

PRESUME

In this book, I would like to introduce you to the therapeutic use of natural herbs, meditation (mind/body power), and a proper nutrition for the cancer prevention and healing. Additionally, I have compiled and provided for your information a short review of some of the most popular alternative cancer therapies.

My only intent, while preparing this guide, was to offer you educational health information that, in my best belief, and best intention, may help you prevent, fight and overcome cancer. However, it is not my intention to directly or indirectly dispense a medical advice or prescribe the use of herbs or food as a form of treatment in lieu or without a medical approval.

Please seek professional help, and take all possible medical treatments, as prescribed by your doctors, and see your doctors regularly. The publisher and author assume no responsibility in the event you use information presented in this guide without your doctor's approval.

To find a doctor who is familiar with natural therapies, you may try to contact the following organizations, which may help you in locating licensed medical professionals in your area (Note: This information may be subject to change).

- American Holistic Medical Association
  2002 Eastlake Avenue East
  Seattle, Washington 98102
  Tel. 206-322-6842

- American Association of Naturopathic Physicians
  PO Box 20386, Seattle, Washington 98102, Tel. 206-323-7610

For more information on herbal medicine, nutrition and alternative treatments, you may read the books listed in the References.

You may also write to the following organizations;

- The American Botanical Council
  PO Box 201660, Austin, Texas
  The Herb Research Foundation
  1007 Pearl Street
  Suite 200, Bolder, Colorado 80302

- Gerson Institute
  PO Box 430
  Bonita, CA 91908
  Tel. 619-472-7450

- International Academy of Holistic Health and Medicine
  218 Avenue B
  Redondo Beach, CA 90277
  Tel.310-540-0564

- International Academy of Nutrition and Preventive Medicine
  PO Box 18433, Asheville, NC 28814, tel.704-258-3243

The following organizations specialize in cancer treatments, involving alternative and complimentary treatments:

- Arlin J. Brown Information Center
  P.O.Box 251
  Fort Bervoir, VA 22060

- Cancer Control Society
  2043 North Berendo Street
  Los Angeles, CA 90027
  Tel. 213-663-7801

- CANHELP
  3111 Paradise Bay Road
  Port Ludlow, WA 98365-9771
  Tel. 206-437-2291

- Center for Advancement in Cancer Education
  300 East Lancaster Avenue

Suite 100, Wynnewood, PA 19096
Phone 215-642-4810

- Foundation for Advancement in Cancer Therapy
P.O.Box 1242
Old Chelsea Station
New York, NY 10113
Tel. 212-741-2790

- The Health Resource
209 Katherine Drive
Conway, AR 72032
Tel. 501-329-5272

- International Association of Cancer Victors and Friends
7740 West Manchester Avenue
Suite 110
Playa del Rey, CA 9029, tel. 213-822-5032

- World Research Foundation
15300 Ventura Boulevard
Suite 405
Sherman Oaks, CA 91403
Tel. 818-907-5483

The key to good health is taking personal responsibility for it. I hope that this book will help to point you in the right direction.

INTRODUCTION

Why did I start my investigation into the cancer disease?

Why did I get at all involved in the field of cancer prevention and natural therapies?

The answer is simple—I wanted to help my husband after he was diagnosed with a metastasized pancreatic cancer. We were told that he had less than a 5% chance to survive longer then two years after his operation.

We were also told by his doctors that if this cancer doesn't come back in a three years' time, my husband would be practically cancer free.

Yes, he was following up on my treatment religiously for the first three years after his operation, leading at the same time a happy and productive life without any treatment in a hospital. He lived a happy life with no pain and fear.

At this time, I started to write this review as a help to other people—not necessarily cancer patients. Maybe, also, to help the spouses or friends of cancer patients—to help them deal with their daily problems and to encourage them to have hope.

For almost four years, there was no sign of a pancreatic cancer coming back—the doctors told my husband that he was cancer free practically and all what he needed was a check-up once a year.

After it, my husband started to express opinion that he never had any pancreatic cancer and his doctors made a mistake in their diagnosis.

Then, he changed his diet and gave up on taking some of the "prescribed" him by me supplements, while still following on only some of the other treatments.

If only I knew about it!

A Guide on Prevention, Natural Healing and Alternative Cancer Therapies

1

KNOW YOUR ENEMY—AN INTRODUCTION TO THE BASIC MECHANISM OF CANCER

What the cancer really is? What causes it? How to fight it?

You have to know more about your enemy. When you know your enemy, its weak side, it is much easier to fight it, isn't? There were many scientific books in this field which I reviewed, and where you can find more scientific and accurate data concerning this disease. If you are interested in more information, you could go to your local library, and look around.

Since I am not a medical scientist, the information that I want to share with you will be a very basic one—just some simple facts.

I found out that according to the findings presented in a medical literature, a majority of cancers is caused by environmental factors—carcinogens such as for example, asbestos, toxic chemicals, air and water pollution, viruses, and electro-magnetic radiation. Additionally, improper nutrition, stress and trauma etc., can contribute to cancer development.

All these factors can cause damage or change in a normal cell, and this cell can become cancerous. Also, the defect can be of a genetic nature, e.g. possession of oncogenes. The genetic code may have an instruction to produce a cancer cell, or the code may become abnormal, due to inherited reasons.

Both environmental factors and genetic defects can cause cancer development.

The damage to a series of genes may cause cells to behave abnormally. According to recent findings, the cells with damaged DNA disregard normal growth constraints, and begin to divide, multiply in number, and then show unrestrained, unregulated growth.

They can also acquire changes in their genes that help them to move freely, enter the circulatory systems win over the immune system and metastasize throughout the body, establishing new growths elsewhere.

The basic mechanism of cancer was explained in a research work of Dr. Otto Warburg, the Nobel Prize laureate. He has discovered that the major difference between normal cells and cancer cells was that the normal cells require oxygen for the energy production, and the cancer cells do not need oxygen to survive.

Both the normal cells and cancer cells use glucose to produce energy. According to Dr. Otto Warburg, if a normal cell is disturbed by a carcinogen, for example a radical, this cell undergoes a change. This change can prevent oxygen from entering a cell, but glucose can enter the cell without any restriction and without presence of oxygen, this glucose is metabolized into a lactic acid.

However, while normal cell produces about 30 energy units for each glucose unit combined with oxygen, the cancer cell produces only 2 energy units. Additionally, cancer cells during this anaerobic (without oxygen) reaction produce a large quantity of "waste" lactic acid. This lactic acid induces an acid environment inside the cell, which in turn causes changes in the DNA of the cell, allowing for uninhibited reproduction of the altered cell. The toxic enzymes produced during this reaction can accelerate the spreading and metastases of cancer cells. The "waste" lactic acid can be converted to glucose again by the liver, and to some extent, by the kidneys.

If cancer develops, and more and more cancer cells show up in the human body, they need more and more glucose for the energy production. They will stimulate the liver and kidneys to produce more glucose from the lactic acid waste. These conditions will also deprive normal cells of the energy source derived from glucose. This creates a devastating state, from which more patients can actually die, then from the cancer itself. It is this uncontrolled multiplication of cancer cells that makes them so malicious, since a growing tumor mass can eventually deprive body's vital organs of nutrients and other energy sources.

Basically, a tumor is a new tissue made of cells that grow without normal restrictions.

Tumors can be either malignant or benign.

Benign tumors are usually not fatal. Malignant tumors grow rapidly and invade surrounding normal cells and spread (metastasize) to other organs within the body, through lymph system and blood vessels.

The basic mechanism and development of cancer involves such stages as:

1. Alteration of a genetic code, activation of oncogenes through carcinogens.

2. Growth of the proliferating cells into cancer, that builds its own blood supply and develops own defense system.

3. Metastasis to other organs.

According to the above findings, arresting of cancer development and stopping it from spreading further can be achieved by arresting new blood vessels' development (angiogenesis), by "starving" them, for example by making the lactic acid conversion to a glucose an impossible one, by changing "pH" (acidity) of cancerous cells into alkaline, and by other means that may include genetic code alteration.

A lot of research is being done on cancer, and billions of dollars are being spent on this research. Consecutively, new developments in treating this decease occur, and we should hope that one day this disease would stop to threaten a human race; cancer will be eliminated, or will be totally treatable.

Let's hope that these officially recognized and scientifically proven treatments will be either similar or possibly based on the natural, alternative therapies so they will be not as abusive to the human bodies as many currently used conventional cancer treatments.

Summary

1. Cancer needs glucose to thrive. Eliminate from your diet such foods as white, refined sugar, ice cream, sodas, cookies, candies, etc., (You can eat instead naturally sweet, dried fruits which provide in a healthy way an adequate quantity of a "natural" glucose needed by the body.)

2. <u>Cancer can develop more easily in the acid environment</u>—when your body's systems pH is low. Switch to the alkaline diet, and consume low in sodium, potassium rich foods (For example, bananas, potatoes, and other potassium rich fruits/vegetables.) Also, coffee (including "90 % acid free "coffee) should be eliminated from your diet!

2

KNOW YOUR FRIEND, THE IMMUNE SYSTEM—THE ROLE OF THE IMMUNE SYSTEM IN CANCER FIGHTING

When you find out that you have an enemy, in most cases you may do two things; either to ignore it, or to fight it. Sometimes, in very rare cases and only if your enemy is intelligent enough; you can try to make friends with it.

However, if either friendship or ignoring your enemy do not work, and your enemy threatens you more and more, your life may become unbearable, and finally, it is a "life or death" situation—your enemy or you.

You have only two choices—either to fight, or to die!

You may decide—" I will see my doctor, and he will kill my enemy—cancer!"

"An operation, followed by some chemotherapy, will kill this cancer and this entire life threatening situation will be over!"

Your enemy will disappear!—Right?

It is only, in many cases, an illusion!

Quite often, one operation is not enough, and your enemy comes back to life—as a matter of fact, it was never killed. At the best, it was "almost" killed. It was killed in one place of your body, but, somehow, it was able to metastasize and spread somewhere else.

Only one tiny particle, one cancerous cell, after traveling within body system, had found a "safe harbor" and is waiting for another opportunity to grow.

It could wait for days, weeks, months or even years—you never know!

And bang! It is back, well, and alive!

"Kill it with chemotherapy," the doctor may say. "Kill it with another operation," he may say. Your enemy, cancer, will be annihilated forever!

Is it true?

In some cases it may be true, but in some other cases it may be only partially true. Each chemotherapy, while killing cancerous cells, may also make some damage to your body's healthy cells. There is no way, according to research findings, that absolutely no damage to the body's healthy parts is made after cancer is attacked by chemotherapy.

Yes, you can have another operation—but how many more?

So, what is the answer? How to fight cancer?

I believe that an answer lays in the following question:

How may I prevent cancer?

How can I prevent it from coming back after operation?

Can I live a normal life as before, eat the same "good stuff" as before (for example, the tasty, fat, barbecued beef steak, with these wonderful French fries, soaked in the overcooked/overheated "vegetable" oil, white bread, and for a desert, a favorite cake, ice cream and coffee?"

The answer is—You may live normal life, as before, but better stay far away from the above "good stuff"! These foods will not provide the proper nutrition to your body!

They will provide some nutrition, for sure, and a lot of calories!

But will they provide a nutrition that will help to make your immune system stronger so you will be more immune to the diseases? Will they make your body strong?

"But, what is it, the immune system?"—you may ask.

It is your friend—a friend that is within your body. This friend, if properly supported, will fight for you, and will defend you!

However, you must take good care of your friend!

It means—you must keep it strong!

"The immune system,"—You may ask again,—"How does it work?"

Again, I want to make it clear that I do not pretend to be an expert in medical sciences.

You may visit your local library, and find a scientific description of the immune system—your biological defense system.

However, for those who "never have time" I have enclosed a short and basic introduction to the immune system which, I hope, can give you some idea, what it is and how works the immune system.

When you get to know your friend better, you will also know how to support friendship!

Basically, according to the medical science findings, the immune system is the organ system that predominantly consists of the spleen, bone marrow, lymph nodes, and lymphoid cells circulating throughout the body. According to the scientists, this system protects the body from harmful foreign substances such as bacteria, viruses, and malignant cells.

The spleen is a large, glandlike immune organ in the abdominal cavity. It is a major site for antibody production. It processes red blood cells and also serves as a blood reservoir.

The lymph is a second circulatory system containing lymphocytes. It flows through all tissues and empties into the blood circulation.

Lymph nodes are bean-sized organs located throughout the body in the route of lymph flow. The immune cells are formed and stored there.

Lymphocytes are cells of the immune system. They are genetically programmed to recognize and bind specific antigens (foreign bodies) and stimulate the development of more lymphocytes reacting with these antigens.

T- and B-cells comprise the two main lymphocyte subpopulations. Lymphocytes are contained in lymphatic organs e.g. in the thymus.

Thymus is a gland-like organ located in the chest. It is mainly responsible for development of T-cells (T-lymphocytes.)

B-Cells (B-lymphocytes) are immune cells derived from bone marrow. They are precursors of plasma cells that produce antibodies to protect against infection. The antibodies (for example immunoglobulin) are produced in response to antigens. Antigens are foreign bodies; viruses, bacteria, toxins, proteins etc.

T-cells (killer cells) are cytotoxic cells that, upon activation by a specific antigen, target and attack the cells bearing that type of antigen.

Macrophages are immune cells that can encompass and digest foreign and toxic matter within the body's tissues. They are helpful in immune cell activation.

According to Norman Cousins, author of the "Head First, The Biology of Hope"/1/, the following can illustrate an action of the body's immune system, for example, against the viruses. It was quoted from the "Nutrition Action Health-Letter", copyright 1988, Center for Science in the Public Interest.

1. Invaders (viruses) enter the body and try to replicate as quickly as possible, before the immune system will organize the defense.

2. Macrophages recognize the invaders as a "foreign threat". They begin to destroy them by flowing to them and enclosing them.

3. Stimulated by the release of interleukins from macrophages, Helper T-cells, and interferon, Natural Killer Cells join the attack on viral infected cells. They can also fight cancer cells.

4. Helper T-cells, start emit signals to immune B-cells and cytotoxic T-cells asking them to join the attack.

5. B-cells, produced in bones, mature into plasma cells, which in turn produce antibodies.

6. Antibodies recognize a particular invader. Then antibodies try to bind to the invader and neutralize it.

7. Cytotoxic T-cells emit lethal proteins on viral infected cells.

8. As the body immune system begins to win, suppresser T-cells help it to slow down. Otherwise, the immune system may attack the body.

9. As the invaders are being defeated, the body creates "memories"; T- and B-cells that circulate permanently in the bloodstream. Next time they will promptly recognize and fight this particular infection.

Summary

You really do not have to remember all this complicated information, such as names and action of each member of the immune system.

It is enough to remember that you have friends in your body. These friends are called "white cells"—lymphocytes. Imagine that each of these lymphocytes carry a sword. These friends are your army. They will fight in your defense, with their swords.

However, they have to be strong!

You have to take care of them! You have to feed them properly!

3

HOW TO STRENGTHEN YOUR IMMUNE SYSTEM

According to the National Cancer Institute findings, there are nearly a million new cases of cancer in the USA every year, and it is a second leading cause of death in young people. The number of cases increases every year.

To prevent this situation, the effectiveness of the human immune system has to be improved. An efficient immune system should kill developing cancer cells before they become a tumor and spread further in the body.

If the immune system doesn't work properly, cancer cells, fungi, viruses, bacteria, can prosper and further decrease body's ability to fight diseases.

According to scientific findings, it is the thymus gland that is mostly responsible for the immune system efficiency.

There are formed and matured T-lymphocytes, cells that fight the diseases, including cancer. The thymus gland produces as many as 26 hormonal substances that defend, repair, and rejuvenate human body. These hormones can control growth of cells, content of sugar in the blood and functioning of white cells, including the T-lymphocytes, and other "natural killer" cells.

To fight the cancer, the body's immune system should be made so efficient that cancer cells will be not able to survive and multiply out of control.

According to the published findings, the strengthening of the thymus can be done through proper nutrition, and by the overall strengthening of the entire body with proper foods, vitamins and minerals. In response, the effectively working thymus gland will produce hormones instructing lymphocytes and other blood cells to attack and kill cancer cells and repair the body.

According to Donald Lepore, author of the "Ultimate Healing System"/7/, the following corrective nutrients can strengthen the thymus gland;

- Glandular Substance: Thymus substance

- Vitamins: Vitamin A (BetaCarotene)
    Vitamin B—Complex
    Niacin
    Pantothenic acid
    - Amino Acids: L-Phenylalanine and Tyrosine
    - Minerals: Potassium and Sodium

- Additionally: Bee Propolis
    Echinacea herb
    Astragalus herb

Also, the thymus gland's functioning is in a great measure affected by person's thoughts and attitude. Positive attitude and thinking will help the thymus gland to become stronger, and thus strengthen the body's immune system.

Summary

The immune system, in order to defend you and function properly, has to be strong!

In order to be strong, your immune system—your army of soldiers, have to be properly nourished. Have you ever heard about a successful army of soldiers that were malnourished and hungry? Remember: "To be or not to be" depends on what you eat!

The malnourished soldiers in your army will be hardly able to drug their feet while in a battle!

Also, the "army "of your immune system has to be in good mood! They have to be sure of their victory! Your mood is their mood! You have to fight! You are their general!

One more thing—your army has to be numerous enough (Ask your doctor about an enlarged "white cells count" number—it shows, that your immune system is fighting, for example, an infection.)

Your body has to be able to make an adequate quantity of the white cells—your soldiers!

So, take good care of your friend—the immune system!

But how the immune system may be improved?

Anytime, at a beginning of an infection, such as a running nose, cold, sometimes fever, the following supplements may be taken:

A bee propolis capsules (1 capsule three times daily), a thymus gland tablets (1 tablet 3 times daily), an Echinacea herb capsules (1 capsule 3 times daily), and sometimes Astragalus herb, in addition to an usual dose of vitamins and minerals (Minimum 1000 mg of Vitamin C, also, zinc supplements are very valuable.)

Also, take the above supplements on a preventive basis, especially, when the "flu" season is approaching. Vegetable soup is a must; variations include chicken, beet, bean, tomato, etc., soups. Always put plenty of carrots, parsley root, leek, celery knob, celery leaves, cabbage and onion to all of these soups and some other "extras" in these soups may include potatoes, veal neck bones, etc.

4

THE MIND/BODY SYSTEM—GOD DOES NOT WANT YOU TO BE SICK!

Nobody can be cured from any disease, until such person is on "good terms" with oneself. A peace of mind, and a state of harmony, first with yourself, and then with an environment around you (this environment include your family, friends, neighbors, etc.) are extremely important to your well being.

I wrote this chapter not to tell you about all "known" facts that are presented in more professional books, but mainly because I wanted to share some inspirational directions. These inspirations originate mostly from my own personal feelings.

I deeply believe that through the self-healing, through taking control over the disease into your "own hands" or, in other words, through using mental power and mind/body interaction, one will have better chance to fight fear. This fear can isolate you from help that is coming from the universe around you; universe that is governed through unknown to us yet laws of God—a help from nature.

The meditation presented below was not intended as a replacement of any other treatments but was provided to supplement them. Generally, I wanted to present in this chapter some mental exercises and useful "hints" that may possibly help not only in healing your body through specially programmed brain exercises but, also, they may help you to achieve internal "spiritual" harmony.

Instead of becoming a victim of a fear and panic you may be able to concentrate on your own well—being. It was not my intention to provide any religious directions or an instruction on any religion. Though I am a Christian, I deeply believe that there is only one God for all people, regardless of their religion.

We all, Muslims, Christians, Jews, Buddhists, etc., are his children—and we all should live together peacefully and try to obey his laws. I believe that God does not want us to fight with each other. I also believe, that God does not want anybody to suffer and be sick—and if properly asked, he may help you to fight the disease.

It was found that many miraculous cases of self-healing have occurred after somebody had shown a strong will and helped the body through the mind power. These phenomena, though they can't be solved on a currently known scientific level, are probably due to several factors that include strengthening of the body's immune system through proper mind exercises, and through achievement of internal "spiritual" harmony.

To start this therapy, think about you as made of two parts; one is real YOU—your spirit that can control your mind.

Your mind should govern your second part—your body.

You—through your mind, though you possibly do not realize it fully, you may possess the power and in most cases, dictate your body, what it should do and how it should act.

You can dictate your body when to stand up, walk, and sit down and, also, you can help it through positive thinking and winning attitude.

There is a double interaction—when your body is hungry, it "alarms" you, so you can take a proper action and make food available to it. When your body is tired, it will signal it to you, so you can put it to rest.

There are so many things to be yet researched and discovered about the mind/body connection and interaction. It is an entire "terra incognita"(Unknown land.) Though so many scientific discoveries were recently made concerning material part of our environment and our bodies, nobody can really define what really is, and how works and reacts the human mind. A lot is yet to be discovered not only about the human body including human brain, but also about spiritual and material sides of the human mind.

What the "mind" really is? Is it, as some scientists want us to believe, just a chain of chemical reactions in the brain? Or is it a "spirit's tool"? If first version is assumed, why these chemical reactions occur, how they are directed and coordinated? By whom? What is really behind human "mind" and "human being's" actions?

Who we are?

Why do we have an ability to think independently?

Why do we feel what we feel?

For what reason?

Why one person can get upset and cry seeing cruel things, wrong—doing by others, unhappiness, war disasters, hungry, injured, suffering children?

Why some people do try to improve the world?

Why other people can be indifferent to miseries of others and some can even enjoy making other people more miserable?

Why one person may become a saint and another may become a criminal?

Why Hitler, the worst "beast" of our century—was so successful in his "operations?"

When animals kill mostly when they are hungry, to feed themselves, Hitler and his Nazi supporters were killing other people, his "brothers and sisters", just for a pleasure of killing them in a crazy "mission" of fulfilling some crazy doctrines. These doctrines were bringing annihilation to Jews, Poles, Gypsies and other nations and races. The stories about the Second World War's wrongdoing by Nazis, which I have heard from my parents, still make me cry.

Why was Hitler so successful and has found so many supporters and why he was able to bring such a terrible disaster and suffering to the human race?

Why, nowadays, there are still some "leaders" in some countries who resemble him so much and who still find supporters for some kind of crazy doctrines calling for supremacy of one nation (or religion) over other nations, etc.?

Why, on the other hand some people, like mother Theresa, devoted their entire lives to helping poor and miserable? What makes a person good or bad?

So many discoveries are yet to be made about human beings; not only about their bodies but, also, about their minds and their mind/body interactions.

However, at this point, we do not need to devote ourselves to the scientific definition of the mind. The main assignment while reading this chapter, is to try to convince yourself that your mind can tell your body that it has a chance to win and that it should fight the disease. That it must fight the disease. That it should win over it.

You must influence your mind to have a winning and positive attitude. Your mind should "imagine" and consequently program the brain to direct the immune system and its white cells to actively and successfully fight and win over their enemies—the cancer cells.

Your mind should imagine and impersonate these white cells as good and brave characters, fighting the bad ones—cancer cells. These good "soldiers" have to win over the bad ones.

Even if you are very sick, weak, and desperate—do not imagine yourself as such, but imagine yourself as being strong, healthy, and doing your favorite activities—going outside, walking, jogging, shopping, playing tennis, swimming or gardening, etc, whatever do you like. When you start thinking about your favorite activities, you will start to believe that you will be able to enjoy them again. In this way, you will be putting your fear and despair away, and you will have a purpose to live and fight for your life. You should believe that you, through your mind, can really help your body systems to become active, and to win over the disease.

If you think that it doesn't make any sense, try to think not only about yourself.

Try to think about others, whom you can help after you are well again—think about other people. Think about your family and friends.

Also, there are so many miserable people that may be in a much worse position than you are, and whom you can help when you get better. There should be a purpose in your life.

You were given your life and you should enjoy it and help others to enjoy their lives. Try to see your life as a "school of living"—a school, which you should pass with the best possible grades. Your illness is one of its lessons. It should turn out to your best.

Remember—"God helps people who help themselves".

To get well, a person must have not only a winning, positive attitude, and think positively. You should heal yourself on an internal, "spiritual" level. This can be achieved if you are in a peace and harmony with yourself and a world around you. Try to avoid negative feelings—instead, fill yourself with friendly ones. Fill yourself with love. Love yourself, and if you want to be loved, start loving others.

See all these good, beautiful things around you. See the beauty of the world that surrounds you—the trees, the flowers, the sky and the river, the lake, the ocean, the mountains. Enjoy it. Appreciate today's conveniences. The human race has achieved so much, especially during this century. Appreciate modern civilization, including developments in a medical field.

Find the goodness in everything that surrounds you; the good always has to win over bad.

Remember that you should always have hope. Things can only turn better, if you believe that they will get better. It is not a false hope. Miracles can happen and have happened.

There is a remarkable book that one can enjoy as a reading material. This is a deeply moving and interesting story based on a personal experience that was written by Harry De Camp—"Special Report—Mind/Body Power"/3/.

He described himself when he was in an incurable, terminal stage of cancer. He was "sentenced" by his doctors as "inoperable", and was sent home "to die". He was advised that he had a very short time, maybe a few weeks, to live. However, to everybody's suprise, he overcame his decease, enjoying a long, healthy, and remarkable life. He wanted to share this miracle with others and wrote a special report about his experience. Try to find and read this book.

It is one of the best written and interesting books I have ever read, based on a real life experience. I am enclosing some of the recommendations based on my review of this book, and in addition, on my personal beliefs:

- Fear and panic are your REAL ENEMIES. Instead of panicking, honestly acknowledge your disease.

- Believe and pray. There are stronger powers in the Universe, than the sickness and disasters. Look into the sky—do you see how well is the Universe organized?

- Do not feel lonely. Imagine yourself as a part of the Universe.

So much research has been devoted and so many scientists worked so hard to discover the material side and the laws of the Universe. Almost everybody wants to know how and when the Universe was created.

Was it made, as many scientists want us to believe, by a chance or in other words, by a "Big Bang"; or was it created by a perpetual, ever existing, living energy, intelligent creative force—the divine intelligence called God? Is the Universe that we inhabit just a foreign, cold space filled with distant stars, located thousands of "light years" apart from us? Or is it our "home" that is filled with a friendly living energy?

Though we can't see this energy, the invisible electromagnetic, or other invisible energy waves may surround us. Since we do not have any special "antennas" to see this energy's waves, it is hard for us to believe in its existence.

Everybody has a tendency to doubt in what can't be seen by one's eyes—not to believe in things that can not be seen or touched. Just imagine what could have happened if working TV or radio sets were suddenly shown to our ancestors. It is possible that they would believe that these appliances were a "black magic", possibly made by "unclear" forces such as witches.

Due to limitations in their knowledge, they wouldn't be able to imagine that these phenomena were actually made possible through a presence of the really existing but invisible to them electromagnetic waves that with the help of electricity can transfer a voice or picture at a very long distance. Similarly, it is very difficult for us to imagine that we may be surrounded by some kind of invisible and undiscovered, yet friendly energy waves.

However, though at this point of development in our civilization, nobody can prove this energy existence; we may try to imagine that we are surrounded by it.

Try to imagine that you are not lonely; this energy or light is everywhere around you. Though it is invisible, it may surround you and be with you. Try to imagine this "invisible light" as a friendly and loving energy that brings you love, peace and harmony that brings you all the goodness the Universe is filled with.

Feel this goodness around you. Good has to win over bad. Harmony and love have to win over despair. Fill yourself with love. Feel the loving light around you. Respond to it. You are not alone. The power of the Creator—the power of God—the ever living, loving force is with you.

It may help you if you properly ask it for a help.

Feel that immense, intelligent and loving force of God, who has organized Universe, who has created it, employing some of the laws that had already been discovered by the people, e.g. the Theory of Relativity, and the laws that are yet not discovered, but maybe one day they will be disclosed.

Think about the Nature around you. Our bodies were created by the Nature, by God's material force. The God, like a father, loves his children. He doesn't want you to be sick. He does not want you to suffer. You should ask Him to help you and to heal you.

- However, you <u>MUST BELIEVE THAT YOU WILL BE HEALED</u>!

You must believe that your sickness, your suffering is not for nothing. It has to be a purpose in it and your suffering will work out for your best benefit.

Think about your life, its purpose. Think about what your life can bring to you and other people around you, when you get better. Think about your life as a universal school that gives you a chance to enrich yourself spiritually through learning from its lessons.

Feel forces of Nature, feel its light and energy, and the power to do good things. You should imagine your healing in your mind and affirm it. Surround yourself in this loving light and peace. Imagine your white cells fighting your enemies—cancer cells. Imagine their victory over cancer. Make these mental pictures many times during the day, so they will be impressed into your subconsience.

You must repeat these exercises over and over again, on a daily basis.

- Take all possible medical treatments, as prescribed by your doctors. See your doctors regularly, and take all medications, and all preventive measures indicated by them.

Doctors, medications, food, natural herbs, proper nutrition etc. were given to you by God. They were given to help your body to get better and help you to fight cancer more successfully.

- While doing all above recommended exercises, simultaneously pray to God, as if you have already been healed. Thank him for your healing! Thank him for his kindness and help! This will help you to affirm your healing and your body should start to behave as if it already was healed. Remember—it is very important that you should trust and believe that you will be healed.

- Do these exercises every day for several weeks until you feel you are healed.

- Tell everybody about your healing and help other people. Affirm them that they too can get healed. Teach them how they should act, teach them to have hope, to love and to see goodness in the world around them.

There is a Bible verse from Isaiah:

"Fear thou not; for I am thy God; I will strengthen thee; yea, I will help thee; yea, I will uphold thee with the right hand of my righteousness". (Isa. 41:10).

Summary

While the purpose of this review was mainly to compile available information and describe a proper diet/nutrition and nutritional supplements for cancer prevention and healing, I also wanted to highlight a very important aspect which I believe is extremely important to any successful therapy.

A proper diet and nutrition that include supplements of herbs, vitamins, and minerals is very important to cancer prevention and treatment. However, it is also my sincere belief that this diet/nutrition may not work adequately, unless a person has a proper mental attitude.

A fear and panic may annihilate most, if not all, beneficial effects of any proper, "life saving," nutrition. I believe that nutritional supplements, to work properly, must be taken by a person who has a proper mental attitude.

This proper mental attitude is as important to well—being as nutritional supplements' taking. The best way to achieve this positive mental attitude is to practice spiritual meditation. In my belief, the best mental meditation can be achieved by spiritual prayers.

There is one God for all people, of all races and beliefs—nobody can claim an "exclusive license" to God. The most important happening is that you should believe in Him. He is all wisdom, goodness, love, and mercy.

He does not want anybody to be sick, or suffer.

Believe that if properly asked, God may help you. However, he has to be asked properly. Most of the people may call his name asking him for some kind of help. There may be many prayers asking Him for some favors at the same time when you beg him for your life. For example, people can ask Him for a proper "Lotto combination" at the same time when you ask for yours or your friend/relative's life.

Possibly, all these prayers may be contradicting each other and may never be heard by Him. You should behave as if you have already obtained your favor.

You should thank Him for yours or your relative/friend's recovery in an advance.

Your spiritual meditation should include more words like "<u>Oh God, thank you for saving my life and making me strong and healthy again. Thank you for your help.</u>" This kind of meditation should help you to obtain a better mental attitude instead of just asking and crying for His help. Maybe God can be sometimes tired of all these crying for help from people who later completely forget about Him?

A few people later remember to tell him "Thank you."

You should thank Him on a daily basis, several times a day—even before you are healed. You may try to "invent "your own meditation relating to God in your own words. Instead of waiting in a fear imagine your white cells fighting cancer cells, while saying these special prayers.

Trying to remember that "<u>God helps people who help themselves,</u>" you should help yourself by having a proper mental attitude! This attitude may be only achieved by special meditation/prayers.

5

CLEAN YOUR BODY SYSTEMS FROM TOXINS—PURIFYING DIET

Imagine a lovely pond, full of clean, clear water. A river is flowing through it—this river has beautiful green banks, and a sandy bottom. Water is so clean in the river and pond, that you can see fishes, even water weeds, at its bottom. The fishes thrive in this clean water, they are strong, and you can even see their joy of life; they jump up from the water once in a while, trying to catch insects in the air.

There was no debris ever "dumped" either in this river or in the pond.

Then imagine another pond. The water in this pond is either standing or there is almost no flow through it. The water in this pond is dark-green and badly smells. There is almost no life in this pond; you can't see any fishes—they died long time ago.

Maybe, as the only form of life, there are some bacteria or some other strangely shaped creatures. They enjoy dirty water—they even thrive in it, at least, for a while. However, sooner or later, even these creatures would die in this dirty water. The repelling odor keeps you far away from this pond.

After a close look, you have found a reason for this smell; you have found why there was no real life in this pond. Debris was dumped into the river and has accumulated inside the pond. With no flow, or with a flow greatly impaired, the pond can't clean itself. The river can't clean itself. More and more debris is being dumped into these waters. After a while, the pond is dead.

Now, what a surprise! Is this just a picture of any pond and river, or is it a picture resembling your body? Yes, the river can resemble your blood system. The pond can resemble your liver, or any other organ. Is your body, your blood, clean and properly oxygenated? Are your organs thriving in it?

Or is your body system becoming like this smelling, dirty pond in which garbage was dumped for a long time?

What is your answer?

Hum, how about another meal consisting of a tasty, fat beef steak or a hamburger, plus French fries cooked in a "vegetable" oil, and as an extra, a creamy cake and a strong coffee with a lot of cream? Can you have it?

Sure that you can, please help yourself! But, only once in a while…An occasional "sinning" and only in moderation may go unnoticed—a fresh rain, growth of new vegetation in a dirty water, may clean a dirty pond; also, a cleansing diet may clean your body systems from poison. But if you keep "dumping" all this good "stuff" into your body without ever cleansing it, after a while it may resemble the above described dirty river and a smelling pond, where all bacteria, viruses, and diseases like cancer, will thrive. At least, they will thrive for a while, until the pond dies.

Remember; cleansing the body systems from toxins and impurities is an important step in maintaining your health, and fighting diseases like cancer.

According to Jethro Kloss, the greatest American herbalist and author of the "Back to Eden"/4/, the cancer can be prevented or cured through combination of the following treatments;

- correct food/nutrition

- proper herbs

- water baths

- massage

- fresh air and sunshine

- exercise

- proper rest

All the above treatments may help in elimination of waste matter and can help purify the entire bloodstream and other body cleansing systems.

The self explanatory description of the influence of the proper nutrition on the body's resistance to diseases was given by Jethro Kloss in his book/4/.He described two patients;

- A woman who had a cancer of the lungs, liver and stomach.

She contacted Jethro Kloss seeking his help; however, it was too late to help her. During the postmortem, it was found that her liver was almost entirely taken by cancer. Both her lungs were invaded and the throat and the stomach were full of cancerous growths in them. She was mulnutrished; her stomach was not retaining any food, and her intestines were shrunken.

Upon inquiries with her family, it was discovered that" her diet were white bread, jellies, jams, soda crackers, and other similar denatured foods".

- The second case was of a man, who's main diet were;" pie, ice cream, iced tea and coffee, white bread, peeled potatoes, denatured, preserved foods, liquor, and tobacco". He didn't want to change his diet even after he was diagnosed with cancer, and he liked to joke that "he was going to have what he wanted while he was alive".

After his death, the postmortem revealed that his bowels were full of cancerous growths. His liver was enlarged and full of tumors. The stomach was full of mucus, and its walls were very dark. His heart was very much enlarged, and after it was opened, a large amount of fat was revealed inside of it.

SUMMARY OF THE CLEANSING DIET

It is very important, that after a person is diagnosed with cancer, his/her first treatment includes proper diet and cleansing of a bloodstream by thoroughly relieving constipation and by making active all organs; skin, lungs, liver, kidneys and bowels. These organs should be kept active all the time!

To relieve constipation, an herbal laxative and enemas are recommended.

For the first 3–14 days (depending on the patient's condition—each treatment should be consulted and approved by the nutritionist!), only unsweetened fruits and fruit juices should be consumed.

Such fruits as apples, cranberries, blueberries, red raspberries, cherries, oranges, grapefruits, lemons, peaches, pears, strawberries (ripe), and avocados are recommended during this cleansing diet period.

Tomatoes are especially beneficial, but they should be eaten alone, not with other fruits. The fruit juices should be made of ONLY ONE FRUIT (fruit juices shouldn't be mixed together); orange, grapefruit, pineapple, lemon or grape juices are especially beneficial.

These fruits juices should be taken separately from each other at different times of the day. Herbal teas should be drunk ALTERNATIVELY with fruit juices; herbal tea should be drunk preferably one hour before drinking a juice.

Do NOT use sugar to sweeten any juice or tea.

Also, the consumption of vegetables and vegetable juices is recommended as very helpful against cancer. The vegetables and vegetable juices SHOULDN'T be taken together (at the same meal) with fruits and fruit juices.

Especially beneficial, during this cleansing period, are beet, and then carrot, celery, cucumber, parsley and lettuce juices.

Vegetable juices can be mixed together with each other.

After a few days of a fruit/vegetable only cleansing diet, an alkaline nourishing diet, consisting of vegetable soups, mashed potatoes, natural brown rice, barley, buckwheat (kasha), lentils, etc., is recommended.

The following vegetables are especially recommended;

- Beets

- Broccoli

- Brussels sprouts

- Cabbage; red, green and Savoy cabbage

- Eggplant

- Carrots

- Cauliflower

Also, such vegetables as corn, green lima beans, garlic, onions, cucumber, radishes, watercress, spinach, squash, kale, asparagus, and peppers are recommended.

- The food should NEVER be cooked in aluminum utensils. The best utensils are made of stainless steel. Use only them!

The proper cancer treatment should also include plenty of fresh air and exercises, if possible, outdoors in sunshine. Use sunscreens, and stay in the high sunshine moderately, according to your condition.

Deep breathing exercises should be performed outdoors and at home.

To keep skin active, frequent warm baths should be taken preferably followed by salt glows. Also, alternative hot and cold applications to liver, stomach, spleen and spine are recommended as well as massage and cold towel rubs.

The rooms in the house should be well ventilated and if possible sunny.

After the cleansing diet, the following diet is recommended;

- Eat fresh, uncooked vegetables daily (two to four cups daily)

- Eat one serving of oatmeal daily; it is an excellent fiber source.

- Stay away from unsaturated oils and from margarine totally. They are harmful.

The best fats are cold pressed olive oil and butter.

- Reduce coffee intake to MAXIMUM one cup daily; drink instead herbal teas.

- DO NOT USE SUGAR—it is, especially cane refined sugar, the WORST possible food for cancer patients.

- There are some indications that consumption of meats should be avoided. However, some persons can feel not well if after a long time of eating meat they are suddenly deprived of it. Generally, a broad range of foods, including lean meats only in moderation and only when desired, can be consumed.

The meats, fish, etc., should be broiled or boiled; <u>do not eat barbecued or fried</u> products.

- Do not use refined, processed rice, flour etc.,—use instead "whole grain" natural products. They are much healthier and they supply a lot of needed natural vitamins and minerals.

SUMMARY

Start your day with an herbal tea (Pau D'Arco and other herbs' extract mixed with water), and a usual portion of food supplements and herbs, as further described in this review.

Next, a good idea is to have an oatmeal (with raisins and banana) and a small sandwich, for a breakfast.

By 10 a.m. you may have your "second breakfast"—for example, full grain rye bread sandwiches.

Try not to buy prepared meats, ham, etc., at the supermarkets. If you badly want them, buy these foods at the small meat stores—generally, they sell meats that have fewer preservatives. Consume these meats very sparingly.

Lunch—either take it from home or eat at the health food restaurant, etc.

Include vegetable soup! Also, a variation of lean meats, fish, with unpeeled potato, ziti, or brown rice, and a vegetable salad as a second helping are recommended.

No coffee, sugar, ice cream, sodas, cookies, etc., consumption is advised.

Red wine may be drunk only occasionally.

6

REVIEW OF VITAMINS AND ANTIOXIDANTS—RECOMM ENDED DOSES

There are many articles being written concerning the role of vitamins and "antioxidants" in cancer prevention and fighting. How these "magic" supplements work? Do they really help?

There is an ongoing research worldwide on the influence of these supplements on a disease fighting and some controversy surrounding them, but most of the experts agree that some of these supplements, in proper quantities, are beneficial against cancer.

To understand the action of an "antioxidant", one has to start with the definition of a "free radical". Simply stating, all matter, including human body, is built of molecules—atoms. Each atom, in addition to positive and neutral elements, has an even number of negative elements—electrons that circulate around positrons and neutrons.

If an atom looses one or more of its electrons, it becomes positively charged; it becomes a "free radical".

This free radical, in an attempt to return to its balanced state, tries to "grab" an electron from another molecule, for example, from the body cell. Thus, damage to this cell can occur, which can cause alteration of this cell's genetic code and can introduce cancerous changes in it.

Carcinogens are substances that are easily becoming "free radicals". One of them is super oxide, a by-product of the oxygen metabolism.

The "antioxidants" are substances that neutralize free radicals by sacrifying themselves.

They sacrifice their electrons to the more aggressive "free radicals", thus becoming free radicals themselves. However, according to the scientists, they are less dangerous to human bodies and in time, they can be converted back to their original condition.

The following nutrients and enzymes, in doses as recommended below/16/, can defend body against free radicals and are therefore called antioxidants;

- <u>Vitamin A and beta-carotene.</u>

To reduce risk of cancer, a daily intake of 5000 to 10000 IU of vitamin A or 25000 to 40000 IU of beta-carotene (precursor of vitamin A) supplement is recommended in the available literature. However, recently there was some warning concerning the vitamin A/betacarotene supplements—they shouldn't be overdosed!

According to the research findings, Vitamin A, among other beneficial functions to the body, can inhibit carcinogenesis, regulate cell development, and strengthen the immune system. According to this review, <u>up to 25000 IU of beta-carotene</u> is adequate.

Vitamin A supplements are more effective if taken with vitamin B complex, vitamins C, D, F, and minerals calcium, phosphorus, and zinc.

- <u>Vitamin C</u>—daily intake of 2000 to 4000 mg is recommended in the available literature.

However, according to this review, <u>a maximum dose of 500-mg of vitamin C daily</u> is sufficient (With exception for cold/flu symptoms when taking of 1000 mg–2000 mg daily for one to three days may be more beneficial.) Synthetic vitamin C is more effective when it is taken with other vitamins, bioflavonoids, calcium and magnesium.

- <u>Vitamin E and selenium</u>—according to the literature, these two substances have synergetic anti-cancerous effect. They should be taken together to give more efficient protection against growth of cancerous tumors.

A daily intake of 400 to 800 IU of vitamin E and 200 (even 400 mcg) micrograms of selenium is recommended in an available literature, as a cancer prevention treatment.

According to this review, <u>a dose of 100 mcg of selenium and 400 IU of vitamin E daily</u> is beneficial.

- <u>Sulfur compounds</u>; according to the research findings, sulfur compounds can increase resistance to cancer. These substances are present in sulfur-rich foods such as garlic.

A lipoic acid, glutathione, n-acetylcysteine, cysteine, cystine and methionine are most important anti-oxidants based on sulfur compounds.

On the basis of my review, I believe that sulfur compounds are available in certain foods (for example, eggs), in adequate quantities and no supplements are needed.

- Trace minerals such as copper (recommended dose 1.5–3 mg), manganese (2–5 mg), and iron (10–15 mg) and especially zinc (15 mg) are important both as components of the antioxidant enzymes and as enhancers of the immune system.

I strongly believe that taking of <u>50 mg to 100 mg of zinc</u> daily is very beneficial

- <u>Vitamin B complex</u>—other important supplements that can offer increased protection against cancer are vitamin B complexes. According to medical research, vitamin B12 and folic acid appears to prevent precancerous growth in cigarette smokers' lungs. (500 mg of vitamin B complex twice a week is recommended.)

- <u>Calcium and vitamin D</u>—according to medical research, dietary supplements of vitamin D and calcium reduce the risk of colon cancer. As a preventive treatment, 800 milligrams of elemental calcium and 200 up to 400 IU of vitamin D are recommended.

- <u>Choline and Dimethylglycine</u>—according to research findings/16/, deficiency of choline can introduce precancerous changes in human body. It is believed that Dimethylglycine strengthens the immune system. The above supplements are available in a properly balanced diet, and in the most of regular multivitamin—multimineral supplements.

- Other nutrients that, according to publications, offer protection against cancer include caretonoids (canthaxantin, lycopene and lutein), found in vegetables and fruits, bioflavonoid (pycnegol, rutin, and quercetin), omega-3 fatty acid EPA (eicosapentaenoic acid) found in cod and water fish, omega-1 fatty acid GLA (gamma-linolenic acid) found in the evening primrose oil, conjugated linoleic acid CLA ellagic acid, found in fruits and nuts, limonene, found in orange peels, epigallocatechin gallate, found in a green tea, and compounds such as dithiolthione, glucarate and sulforaphane, found in cruciferous vegetables of a "cabbage family."

SUMMARY

I believe that a properly balanced diet already provides several of the above listed vitamins, minerals, etc.

Basically, the following vitamins and minerals supplements, while taken on a daily basis, in the following daily doses are beneficial:

- Betacarotene—25,000 IU

- Vitamin C—500 mg

- Vitamin E—400 IU

- Selenium—100 mcg

- Zinc (Gluconate)—100 mg

- Potassium (Gluconate)—500–1000 mg (min. 83.5 mg content)

- Multivitamin/Multimineral supplément—1 capsule

7

"TO BE OR NOT TO BE "DEPENDS ON WHAT YOU EAT

You may wish to skip this chapter if you think that you are already an expert on this topic. As I have already stated it previously, the proper cancer preventive and fighting diet should include more fruits and vegetables, more whole grains and eventually lean meat, including fish.

Less of heavy meats, dairy foods, and prepared and packaged foods should be consumed. Smoked and salt cured foods should be avoided. According to many experts, a diet high in fat can make a person more vulnerable to cancer.

Do you know that according to the research at the National Cancer Institute in Bethesda, Maryland, 35 percent of ALL cancers are linked to high-fat diets?

Oliver Alabaster MD, Director of the Cancer Research at the George Washington University in Washington, DC indicated that there is evidence that 60 percent of all cancers in women and 40 percent of all cancers in men are caused by a wrong diet.

American Cancer Society guidelines recommend limiting of fat intake to 30% of total calories, but several experts say that fat intake should be further reduced to 20% of all calories. According to James O'Brien, author of the "Foods That Fight Cancer/10/, low-fat diet reduced the blood levels of the hormone estradial, in women which were put on a low fat diet in the experiment performed at the Fred Hutchinson Cancer Center in Seattle. This hormone is a form of estrogen that has been connected to breast cancer occurrence.

As prevention, the fat intake in an average calories intake of between 1,600 to 2,400 calories a day should be less than 50 grams daily (preferably up to 35 grams of fat a day). However, the body also needs some fat and proteins to function, and these nutrients should not be eliminated completely from the diet.

According to many experts, the best source of fat is a cold pressed olive oil that is abundant in monosatured fat content. You may also use canola oil for cooking.

Additionally, an olive oil also helps to control "bad" cholesterol level.

The worst possible fats are margarine and unsaturated fats (e.g. corn oil, etc.) and should be avoided.

FRUITS AND VEGETABLES

Everybody knows already that the consumption of fruits and vegetables helps fight and prevent cancer. The fruits are not only fat free, have fiber, but at the same time they are rich in essential vitamins and minerals. Especially, they are rich in natural antioxidants, and they also contain thousands of Cancer-retarding substances called phytochemicals.

The primary antioxidants present in the fruits are vitamins A, C, E and trace mineral selenium.

The vitamins, antioxidants and phytochemicals provided in daily servings of fresh fruits and vegetables are much more beneficial and easier absorbed in human bodies than these available in synthetic versions.

The most recognized at present phytochemicals are sulforaphane (broccoli, cauli-flower), indole-3-carbinol (cabbage, cauliflower), allylic sulfide (onion, garlic), capsaicin (hot peppers, turmeric, and cumin), flavonoids (present in almost every vegetable and fruit), p-coumaric and chlorogenic acids (tomatoes), phenethyl isiothiocyanate GPE (TC) (Available in broccoli, cabbage, and turnips), genistein (soy beans.)

These substances fight harmful components such as free radicals.

By eating fruits and vegetables rich in antioxidants one can substantially reduce the risk of cancer. Two to four servings of fruits and vegetables a day are recommended by most nutritionists.

For example, the average serving of fruit provides between 80 to 120 calories, approximately 25 grams of carbohydrates, 1 gram of protein and 3 to 4 grams of fiber.

Additionally, about 1000 IU of Vitamin A and 30 to 60 grams of vitamin C are provided with average fruit serving/10/.

The cancer fighting fruits can be divided into 2 groups;

- Vitamin A (Betacarotene) fruits

- Vitamin C fruits

Below, I provided a basic review of these fruits and vegetables, for your information.

VITAMIN A FRUITS

The vitamin A fruits provide alpha-, beta-and other carotenes. The plant form of vitamin A is more beneficial and easier absorbed by the liver, than animal based vitamin A.

According to tests performed at the National Cancer Institute, an adequate supply of vitamin A can reduce the chance of certain cancers for about 30 to 50 percent.

It was discovered, that carotenes, especially alpha- and then beta-carotene, among other beneficial functions to the body, inhibit carcinogenesis, regulate cell development, and strengthen the immune system.

Most of vitamin A/carotene rich fruits and vegetables have a pulp that has orange, yellow or red colors.

If synthetic supplements of vitamin A are taken, they are more effective when taken with vitamin B complex, vitamins C, D, F, and minerals calcium, phosphorus, zinc.

The following fruits are rich in vitamin A;

- MANGOES

- PAPAYAS

- APRICOTS

- PEACHES

- PRUNES

- WATERMELON (Watermelon should be eaten separately, from other meals.)

- NECTARINES

- CANTALOUPES

- HONEYDEW

VITAMIN C FRUITS

It have been observed, that people who have diets rich in vitamin C, have higher rate of protection against cancer.

Similarly like beta-carotene, it is a strong antioxidant. It can prevent free radicals built-up inside the body as well as destroy them. It also can neutralize preservatives found in a cured, preserved and luncheon meat.

These chemical compounds; e.g. nitrates and nitrites, react with the compounds in the body such as amines, thus forming powerful carcinogens such as nitrasamines.

Also, vitamin C can strengthen the immune system and increase its resistance to some infections. According to the research findings, vitamin C also enhances built-up of a collagen inside the body; collagen in turn can help the body to fight against the cancer. When tumor starts to grow, the immune system can encapsulate the growth with the collagen and stop it from further spreading.

Though the cancer cells try to neutralize and dissolve the collagen walls with enzyme called hyaluronidase, the vitamin C can also counteract hyauronidase action.

The recommended daily allowance of vitamin C is 60 mg, however, according to many experts; 1000 mg (1 gram) to 2000 mg daily can provide more effective cancer protection.

Since it is difficult to achieve such levels of vitamin C with fruit diet alone, taking of supplements can be necessary.

Synthetic vitamin C is more effective when taken with other vitamins, bioflavonoids, calcium and magnesium. Too much of vitamin C will displace sulfur level, so an adequate supply of sulfur (available in eggs), should be assured. Also, the cigarette smoking reduces level of vitamin C in the body (Each cigarette uses up to 25 mg of vitamin C.)

The fruits rich in vitamin C are;

- GUAVA

- CURRANTS

- KIWIFRUIT

- GRAPEFRUIT

- MANGOES

- LEMONS

- ORANGES

- STRAWBERRIES

- TANGERINES

- RASPBERRIES

- BLACKBERRIES

VEGETABLES

According to numerous published articles, the deep green and deep yellow vegetables are the most powerful foods against cancer—they contain compounds called indoles which have ability to prevent tumor growth.

These vegetables also contain beta-carotene and vitamins C, E, B and cancer inhibiting trace mineral selenium.

Similarly like fruits, there are vitamin A vegetables, vitamin C vegetables and "cabbage family" vegetables.

Vitamin A rich vegetables are;

- BEETS AND BEET GREENS

- CARROTS

- KALE

- SPINACH

- SQUASH (winter).

- SWEET POTATO

- TURNIP GREENS

- ENDIVE

- BLACK-EYED PEAS

- CORN

- ROMAN LETTUCE

- SQUASH (summer)

- SOYBEANS

- PEPPERS (bell)

- TOMATOES

Unlike vitamin A and B complex, the cooking can destroy vitamin C, so these vegetables should be eaten raw, for example with a dressing etc.

Vitamin C rich vegetables are;

- COLLARDS

- PARSLEY

- ASPARAGUS

CABBAGE FAMILY VEGETABLES

Cabbage family vegetables are also called "cruciferous" vegetables. These vegetables have special cancer fighting properties; they contain chemicals called "indoles" and "aromatic isthiocyanates". These compounds keep normal, healthy cells from turning cancerous, and from uncontrolled growth, as well as they can block a promotion of cancer.

Also, the cabbage family vegetables have special enzyme-inducer chemicals. These chemicals stimulate the body to produce enzymes that protect its cells against cancer growths.

These vegetables are also rich in vitamin A, calcium and selenium.

According to James O'Brien, a research study has revealed that people who ate raw vegetables, especially broccoli, cauliflower, and cabbage, had as much as 3 times less chance to develop a colon cancer and much less chance to develop a stomach cancer. People on brussel sprouts and cabbage diet have shown an ability to break faster test carcinogens, than people on normal diet.

The National Academy of Sciences Committee on Diet, Nutrition, and Cancer has confirmed special cancer fighting properties of the cabbage family vegetables.

The following vegetables have these abilities;

- BROCCOLI—one cup contains about 1355 IU of vitamin A, 80 mg of vitamin C, plus calcium, indoles, aromatic isothiocyanates, and enzyme promoters.

- CABBAGE (Savoy)—one cup of cooked vegetable provides about 1300 IU of vitamin A and 25 mg of vitamin C.

- BRUSSELS SPROUTS—1 cup provides about 1,120 IU of vitamin A, 95 mg of vitamin C, plus indoles, protein, iron, potassium and fiber.

- CABBAGE (green)—1 cup of shredded cabbage provides about 90 IU of vitamin A, 25 mg of vitamin C, and some potassium and calcium.

- CABBAGE (red)—has about 30 IU of vitamin A, and 40 mg of vitamin C.

- CAULIFLOWER—1 cup provides about 70 mg of vitamin C.

According to Earl Mindell, author of the "Herb Bible"/9/, the National Cancer Institute is currently investigating several concentrated plant compounds to be used in foods that will help to prevent and fight cancer. These "designer foods" will contain plant compounds, including indoles from cabbage family and other anticarcinogenic plant chemicals.

It is possible that in the future there will be a cereal designed especially for women with breast cancer risk and another one for people at risk of colon cancer, etc.

The delicious recipes with possible cancer curative power are available in "The Healing Foods Cookbook"/14/.

FISH AND FISH OIL

The studies in Canada have shown that fish oil reduces the rate of breast cancer. Researches have found that omega-3 fatty acids boost the body immune system, thus preventing tumor formation, and help destroy developing tumors. The following fish are high in polyunsaturated fat, that can reduce breast cancer risk;

- SALMON—about 155 calories in 3 ounces

- TUNA—about 110 calories, per 3 ounces (tuna in water)

The following fish are rich in omega-3 acids;

- MACKEREL—has about 175 calories per 3 ounces

- SARDINES—has about 135 calories per 3 ounces

Most of the fishes can provide a delicious, low-calorie meal, and secure necessary protein supply. The fish shouldn't be cooked or broiled in butter; instead, cook it in a wine with lemon and herbs to flavor.

LEAN MEATS

Most of the meats have high fat content, and preferably they should be avoided, or seldom consumed. The following meats can provide low fat meals;

- TURKEY—has about 155 calories per 3 ounces

- CHICKEN (should be prepared/eaten without skin!)—About 130 calories per 3 ounces (white meat); 23 % of them from fat. 175 calories (dark meat); 30% of them from fat.

- LEAN VEAL—contains about 185 calories per 3 ounces (30 % fat)

- TOP ROUND—about 165 calories (20 % fat) per 3 ounces

- EYE OF ROUND—has about 170 calories (33% fat) per 3 ounces.

8

"AND THE LEAVES OF THE TREES WERE FOR THE HEALING OF NATIONS"—A REVIEW OF HERBAL THERAPY

While doing my research on alternative cancer treatments, I have found numerous opinions stating that most of the herbs can be safely used as a therapeutic medicine, with no side effects, for a variety of ailments, including cancer.

What are the herbs?—In the past herbs were defined as flowering plants that die after flowering. However, today an herb is defined as any growing plant, including trees and mushrooms.

The people discovered and utilized the healing abilities of herbs long time ago.

First written descriptions of healing properties of the herb Dittany date to almost 5000 years ago. Herbs Caraway, Laurel and Thyme were also in use in ancient Mesopotamia. About 2700 BC the Chinese wrote a book, on uses, with descriptions, of 365 healing plants. Also, the ancient Egyptians and Greeks used food seasonings, cosmetics and medicines made from herbs.

The Bible says; "And the leaves of the trees were for the healing of nations". Revelation 22:2. Today, chemical drugs mostly dominate the medicine. It is true that these synthetic drugs have the ability to quickly remove the symptoms of illness, and are often life saving.

However, in many situations, these drugs possibly do not treat the real cause of illness, but only relieve its symptoms/6/.

The illness that is not cured can repeat itself or emerge somewhere else in the body, quite often with more serious symptoms. Also, many of the chemical drugs can have adverse side effects. Sometimes, especially if overused, they can create more danger, then the disease, they were supposed to heal.

You can learn about these drugs side effects from such references as for example, "Physician's Desk Reference Book".

However, there are also numerous beneficial synthetic drugs based on extracts from plants. Almost 40% of today's medicine drugs are being derived from plants. For example, one of the most popular medicines today, an aspirin, was discovered and manufactured by chemist Frederick Bayer. He investigated the organic compounds obtained from plants/willow bark/that reduced pain and fever. Then he originated the synthetic compound—acetyl-salicylic-acid, known today as the Bayer's Aspirin.

One of the most recognized recently ovarian cancer treatment drug "Taxol" was extracted from the Pacific Yew tree. This drug has already saved lives of many ovarian cancer patients, and is considered as a very effective medication.

The herbs as medical treatment are probably in highest esteem between Chinese people.

Herbal medicine in China has developed thousand of years ago and there are now over 8,000 herbs in use.

The Chinese medicine puts even more pressure on the prevention and maintenance of health, than on the disease treatment. In the past, Chinese doctors were paid only as long as their patients remained healthy.

The doctors, whose patients were becoming frequently ill, were not regarded as good practitioners.

Their knowledge and abilities were questioned, and they were loosing their clients.

The Chinese consider a human being as impersonation of a living energy. They believe that the energy changes into different forms as it moves, and knowledge of this energy flow (Wu Li) enables predicting and controlling it.

They use herbs to assure a healthy flow of energy, and they believe that several herbs used in combination can give better results than benefit obtained from each herb alone. The combination of primary herb (used for the main purpose) and several secondary herbs (enhancing the effect, directing the flow and reducing side effects etc.) are usually recommended in Chinese medicine, as more effective medical treatment.

There are several herbal combinations recommended by several reputable herbal experts as effective against cancer and tumors.

A review of some of these combinations is presented below. Please note that though these combinations sometimes different from each other, certain/primary/herbs are repeated in them.

- The following herbs are believed as especially beneficial against cancer/11/;

- Chaparral*

- Chickweed

- Dandelion

- Eucalyptus

- Garlic

- Ginseng

- Golden Seal

- Irish Moss

- Parsley

- Poke Weed

- Red Clover*

- Slippery Elm

- Taheebo (Pau D'Arco)*

- Yellow Dock

• Herbs marked with asterisk are considered as most effective against cancer.

The following herbs are considered to be most effective against tumor growths/11/;

- Chaparral*

- Chickweed

- Lobelia

- Mullein

- Plantain

- Poke Weed

- Red Clover*

- Taheebo (Pau D'Arco)*

- Yellow Dock

One of the most recognized pioneers in herbal healing, **Jethro Kloss**, author of the book "Back to Eden"/4/, **recommended the following herbs as the most efficient** in cancer fighting;

- Chaparral

- Echinacea

- Red Clover

- Blue Violet (the whole plant)

- Golden Seal root

- Gum Myrth

- Aloes

- Blue Flag

- Gravel Root

- Bloodroot

- Dandelion root

- African Cayenne

- Chickweed

- Agrimony

- Oregon Grape

- Rock Rose

- Fo-Ti (Ho Shou Wu)

According to Jethro Kloss, the following herbs may be also taken internally for tumor growths, singly and/or in combination of two or three;

- Bayberry

- Slippery Elm

- Mugwort

- White Pond Lily

- Chickweed

- Sage

- Wild Yam

SAGE AND SLIPPERY ELM POULTICES are especially effective against external tumors.

According to Jason Winters, author of the book "Killing Cancer"/18/the following herbal combination, called by him Tribalene, has saved his life;

- Chaparral

- Red Clover

- Herbaline; a special spice from Southeast Asia

Additionally, one 500 mg Amygdalin/Laetrile; Vit. B-17/tablet after three pancreatic enzyme tablets, thirty minutes before each meal were recommended in the above treatment (Amygdalin, according to certain studies, has a very controversial benefit. so check with your nutritionist before starting to take it).

According to Humbart Santillo, ND. author of the book "Natural Healing with Herbs"/12/, the following herbal combination is especially beneficial against cancer;

- Red Clover

- Echinacea

- Chaparral

- Violet Leaves

- Bloodroot

- Dandelion Root

- Santicle

- Buckhorn bark

- Burdock root

- Ginger

- Licorice root

These herbs should be powdered and mixed together in equal parts, and put in no. 00 capsules. Take two capsules four to six times daily.

Along with this combination, garlic, wheatgrass juice and beet juice should be drunk daily. If pain is present, a Wild Yam and Valerian tincture, ten drops every hour, may be applied.

The following combination of herbs was present in Harry Hoxsey therapy:

- Against external cancers, a special paste, made of bloodroot herb, mixed with zinc chloride and antimony sulfide.

- Against internal tumors, a special internal tonic made of basic ingredients such as potassium iodide, and such herbs as licorice, red clover, burdock root, stillingia root, barberis root, pokeroot, cascara, prickly ash bark, and buckthorn bark.

Essiac, a special herbal tea, according to Canadian nurse Rene Caisse, has caused remissions in thousands of cancer patients. The following principal herbs are included in the Essiac combination;

- Burdock root

- Turkey rhubarb root (Indian rhubarb)

- Sheep sorrel

- Slippery elm bark

According to sister Caisse observations made on cancer patients, many patients reported an enlarging and hardening of the tumor after a few treatments. Then the tumor should start to soften and a discharge of puss and fleshy material (in patients with breast, rectal and other internal cancers), may be observed. After this process, the tumor would be gone. Even if a tumor didn't disappear, Caisse maintained, it was forced into regress, and after six to eight Essiac treatments could be removed with much less risk of metastasizing.

To prevent a reoccurrence of cancer, Essiac should be then given at least once a week.

You may try to obtain more information on Essiac at the following address (subject to verification):

Elaine Alexander

HELP NATURE TO HEAL YOU FROM CANCER

6690 Oak Street

Vancouver, British Columbia V6P 3Z2, Canada

Tel. 604-261-1270

Summary

According to this review, the following herbal combination is beneficial:

- Three red clover capsules (in powdered form), three times daily

- An extract made mainly of Pau D'Arco bark (Take at least one standard box of Pau D'Arco tea, in a loose form, or twenty four small tea packets for each glass container of a quarter gallon size of Bacardi rum as a base for this extract, store for three weeks while shaking twice daily.) Drink one to two tablespoons of this extract three times daily.

- In addition, take one capsules each of Echinacea, Dandelion and Slippery Elm Bark herbs, in a powdered form, once daily.

In addition, once daily, other nutritional supplements, such as 100 mcg of selenium, 200 IU of Vitamin E, 50 to 100mcg of zinc, 500 mg of Vitamin C, 25,000 IU of beta-carotene, and one standard tablet of a multivitamin/multimineral formula shall be taken.

Also, drink two to three cups of beet juice daily.

HERBS HELPFULL AFTER CHEMOTHERAPY AND RADIATION

According to herbal experts, the following herbs can have healing effects and may reverse damaging effects of radiation and chemotherapy;

- ASTRAGALUS; according to Earl Mindell, recent studies presented in eminent medical publications in China suggest beneficial influence of Astragalus herb against cancer.

Astragalus may help to activate the immune system and prevent the spread of malignant cancer cells to the healthy tissue.

The research performed at the University of Texas in Houston by Dr. G. Mavligit, has confirmed that an extract from Astragalus had helped to restore normal immune function in cancer patients with impaired immunity/9/.

Astragalus is routinely given by some herbalists to people undergoing chemotherapy and radiation.

Application—Astragalus herb combination "Resist All", during an outbreak of a high fever during recovery period after the operation is recommended.

- ALOE VERA; is especially beneficial for people undergoing radiation treatment. It has been used successfully in the United States for treatment of radiation burns.

External applications of Aloe Vera gel speed healing of external burns and scars—according to research presented in the Journal of Dermatological Surgery and Oncology, the Aloe Vera significantly speeded healing of patients whose top layers of skin were removed through facial dermabrasion/9/.

Application—take Aloe Vera gel (only 97 to 99 percent pure Aloe Vera in liquid form is recommended) internally to heal internal radiation burns, at the end of radiation treatment

- ECHINACEA; this herb is called a "King of Blood Purifiers". It raises the immunity level of the body.

Echinacea has been used to help restore normal immune function in patients receiving chemotherapy.

Application—take Echinacea herb during recovery period, and take one tablet on a daily basis, with the dose increased to three tablets when any sign of cold or other infection is present.

CYSTEINE-According to Dr. Donsbach, an amino acid cysteine (Cysteine Hydrochloride) may protect against radiation damages/2/.

Application—one cysteine tablet three times daily at the end of the radiation treatment.

HERBS HELPFUL AGAINST BREAST TUMORS

Described below treatment was recommended by Humbardt Santillo ND/12/. According to this nutritionist, the breast tumors can be treated both internally and externally; 1. Internal therapy through blood purification can be achieved by drinking herbal teas.

- Drink Red Clover, Sassafras, Chickweed and Burdock root teas. The Red Clover combination capsules carried by Nature's Way products should also be used; take four tablets three times daily

- Take up to five tablets of homeopathic silica (first 4x, then 12x) five times daily. Silica can be excellent against all tumors caused by toxic lymphatic system.

- To keep iodine level of blood normal, take Kelp or Dulse capsules daily.

- Use low sodium, high potassium diets (See chapter on foods.)

- Use Chlorophyll enema implants (wheat grass or parsley juice). Drink two to four ounces of liquid chlorophyll juice, mixed with water or celery or apple juice, two times daily.

2. Together with internal therapy, apply externally any of the following poultices (they may be used alternatively);

- POKE WEED POLTICE (see poke weed, Herb List chapter)

- SOOTHING POLTICE made from equal parts of powdered plantain leaves, comfrey leaves, and lobelia. Mix these leaves with wheat germ and castor oil to a thick consistency. Spread it 1/4 inch thick on linen, and apply to the tumor. Keep it on from four to six hours daily.

- SAGE AND SLIPPERY ELM POLTICE made from equal parts of powdered herbs mixed with water.

- ICHTHAMMOL AND VEGETABLE GLYCERIN POLTICE made from equal parts of mixed together components (Ichtammol can be found in drug stores.)

- POLTICE made of clay, macerated cabbage leaves, flaxseed and a pinch of cayenne.

Mix these ingredients with water spread on linen and apply for several hours.

- THE PULP FROM PRICKLY PEAR CACTUS (Optunia Species) is very helpful on sore, swollen breasts.

To arrest the growth of tumor mass, taking of bovine cartilage is recommended see chapter on alternative treatments.

According to Humbardt Santillo ND, the tumor can get larger at the beginning of the detoxification process—however, once the blood is purified, the tumor should shrink/12/.

Anne E. Frahm, a former "terminal" breast cancer patient/19/recommends the following nutrients, on basis of her personal experience;

- Vitamins: A, beta-carotene, B-Complex vitamins, vitamin C, vitamin E (Emulsified.)—Minerals: selenium, zinc, magnesium, copper

- Additional supplements: EPA-DHA (fish oil), glutathione, Melaleucea Oil, garlic (in form of extract KYOLIC), desiccated liver, pancreatic enzymes, "green drink"(Kyo—Green brand; a blend of green barley, wheat grass, kelp, brown rice and chlorella).

- Also, a high fiber, vegetarian diet is recommended.

PROPERTIES AND LIST OF HEALING HERBS

There are many herbs that are listed by several reputable herbal experts as useful against cancer. Basic information about these herbs' properties is compiled below.

Do not take all these herbs, at once, and on a daily basis. Only a few of these herbs, which are basic herbs, should be taken

From time to time, on as needed basis, take other herbs, as described in this guide.

ALFALFA (Medicago Sativa)

Alfalfa contains vitamin A (beta-carotene), E, K, D, B6 and H. It is very rich in minerals such as calcium, phosphorus, iron, magnesium, silicon, sodium and potassium. It contains 2 potassium units per 1 sodium unit. It has 8 digestive enzymes. It can be taken 3 times daily, before meals. Every two weeks, take two Alfalfa tablets on a daily basis, for a one-week time. (In the evening.)

ALOE VERA (Aloe Barbadenis)

Aloe Vera contains calcium, iron, lecithin, manganese, potassium, and sodium. Also, it contains alocutin A, germanium, and gamma-linoleic acid.

Aloe Vera liquid gel taken internally will help to heal tissues damaged by cobalt radiation. Aloe Vera applied externally will heal X-ray burns, and it is frequently applied after surgery, to speed healing and minimize scars left after incision.

Drink Aloe Vera juice at the end of the radiation treatment.

ASTRAGALUS (Astragalus Membranaceous)

Recent studies in leading medical journals suggest that Astragalus activates the immune system and helps to fight diseases, thus helping against cancer. It contains a bioflavonoid quercitin, polysaccharides, choline, folic acid and betaine.

Oriental herbalists have used Astragalus for centuries for variety of ailments.

Do not take Astragalus herb on a daily basis (An herbal combination that includes Astragalus during high fever period may be beneficial.)

BARBERRY (Berberis Vulgaris)

Barberry contains compounds berberine and oxyacanthine that were found to be active against several cancers, and Barberry is believed to be especially helpful against cancers of stomach, neck and liver.

BEE POLLEN

1000 mg of bee pollen contains 600 mg of natural potassium. Bee pollen is very rich in B-vitamins (B1, B2, B3, B5, B6, and B12).

It also contains vitamins A, C, E, folic Acid, and 20% of its content is proteins and amino acids.

Pollen is a male element of the flower. Only the entomophile pollen (gathered by bees) should be used—the bees recognize which pollens are of the best quality and most nutritious, and thus ensure high quality of the pollen.

Take 500 mg of bee pollen on a daily basis.

BEE PROPOLIS

The Propolis is collected by bees from the resinous substance from buds of trees e.g. horse chestnut, or from cracks in the bark of conifer trees e.g. spruce. According to experts, it is a natural antibiotic.

Its antibiotic properties are believed to come from the flavoids it contains, especially from the galangin.

Propolis is an immune system regenerator and has the ability to strengthen the thymus gland that is responsible for body's immune system.

Propolis is also rich in vitamins B, E, C, H, P, and provitamin A, and it contains trace minerals such as iron, manganese, zinc and others.

It also contains fats, aminoacids, organic matter, and composite ethers of univalent alcohols; cinnamic acid's, cinnamyl alcohol, vanillin, chrysin, galangin, pinostrobin, acacetin, kaempferid, ramnocitrin, caffeic acid, tetochrysin, isalpinin, pinocembrin and ferulic acid/7/.

Take Bee Propolis capsules (one to three daily), during "high risk" flu season, or when you experience any infection.

The Bee Propolis ointment may help to heal difficult to heal wounds, infected after the operation.

BLACK WALNUT (Juglans Nigra)

Black walnut is rich in manganese, iodine, and vit. B15. It also contains potassium, silica, magnesium, calcium, phosphorus, iron and protein. According to research findings, its compounds ellagic acid and juglone show anti-cancer properties. It is believed to be especially beneficial against stomach, thyroid, lymphoma, esophagus and breast cancers.

Black walnut oxygenates the blood to destroy parasites.

BLUE VIOLET (Violet; Viola Odorata)

As a tea, violet leaves will purify the blood. They are also very beneficial in healing of ulcers. For cancerous growths, violet is especially beneficial when combined with Red Clover and Vervain/4/.

BUCKTHORN BUCK (Rhamnus Trangula)

According to research findings, Buckthorn contains aloe-e modin that is active against lymphocyte leukemia, and other cancers. Freshly cut bark shouldn't be used; only the bark that has been dried for over 2 years is recommended.

Buckthorn Bark is also very good as a laxative, and can act as a cleaning agent by keeping bowels regulated.

BURDOCK ROOT (Arctium Appa)

Burdock is one of best blood purifiers. Burdock root contains inulin, mucilage, sugar, lappin resin, fixed and volatile oil, and tannic acid. It is also rich in vitamin C and iron. It also contains vitamins A, B-complex, E, P, and PABA and minerals sulfur, silicon, potassium, copper, iodine and zinc. Burdock is believed to be especially beneficial against digestive organs, lymph glands, and uterus and breast cancers.

Burdock can help adjust hormone balance in the body by nourishing hypothalamus and pituitary glands/7/.

CASCARA SAGRADA (Rhamnus Purshiana)

Cascara Sagrada contains B complex, calcium, potassium, manganese, and traces of tin, lead, strontium, and aluminum, and chrosophanic acid. It contains aloe-emodin that was found to be active against cancers lymhocytic leukemia and Walker carcinosarcoma/22/.

It is a mild laxative, and by promoting bowel function, it can help clean the body systems.

CHAPARRAL (Larrea Tridentata)

The American pioneers learned about this herb from Native Americans. Chaparral is rich in potassium and sodium. It also has silicon, tin, aluminum, sulfur, molybdenum, chlorine and barium.

It is possibly one of best natural antibiotics, which can be used both internally and externally.

Chaparral contains a powerful antioxidant NDGA (nordihydroguiaretic acid). This antioxidant can inhibit the formation of dangerous substances such as free radicals.

Chaparral can prevent the growth of certain cancerous tumors, and can be especially beneficial against such cancers as malignant melanoma, choriocarcinoma, lymphosarcoma, and possibly leukemia.

It purifies the blood from toxic impurities/7, 9/.

CAUTION!!!—This herb shouldn't be used by people with digestive system problems such as e.g. ulcers. While used for a prolonged period of time in excessive quantities it may cause liver disease. Currently, due to the F.D.A restriction, this herb is not available in the health food stores in USA. Instead, an herbal combination "Chaparr-ALL" that has similar properties, or possibly, a sage herb, is recommended.

CHICKWEED (Stelaria Media)

Chickweed is rich in vitamins A, B complex, C, and D. It contains iron, copper, calcium, sodium and traces of manganese, phosphorus, zinc and molybdenum.

Chickweed leaves have a resin and assorted glycosides that have antibiotic properties and can act as antidotes to blood poisoning.

It has also been recommended as anticancer agent.

DANDELION ROOT (Taraxum Officinale)

Dandelion root enhances and strengthens liver and gallbladder functions, and also has water removing and detoxifying properties. Dandelion is believed to be especially beneficial against bowel, bladder and breast cancers. It is rich in inuline, a substance helpful to kidneys and pancreas.

Dandelion contains vitamins A, B, C and E, is rich in potassium, and contains calcium, sodium, phosphorus, iron, nickel, cobalt, tin, copper, zinc and substances taraxerol, choline, levulin, inulin and pectin. It also has a lecithin, a substance that may protect against cirrhosis of liver/7, 9/.

ECHINACEA (Echinacea Augusti Folia)

This herb was introduced first by Native Americans. Echinacea has positive effect on the immune system. Studies have shown that echinacin B, a compound of Echinacea prevents the formation of an enzyme called hyaluronidase, which destroys a natural barrier between healthy tissue and unwanted pathogenic organisms. A study presented in The Journal of Medical Chemistry, in 1972, has shown that Echinacea extract has inhibited tumor growth in rats.

According to recent research findings, oil extracted from roots of Echinacea is active against cancers lymphocyte leukemia and Walker's carcinoma.

Echinacea stimulates the lymphatic system and raises the blood cell count in the body.

Echinacea contains vitamins A, C, and E, and minerals iron, iodine, copper, sulfur, and potassium. It also has inulin, sucrose, betain, echinacein, myristic acid, echinacosideresins and various fatty acids.

Both betaine and echinacoside are cells manipulators and help heal certain forms of cancer/7/.

Take Echinacea herb during "high risk" flu season, or when you experience an infection.

EVENING PRIMROSE (Oenothera biennis)

Evening primrose oil is believed to be beneficial against benign breast diseases. According to research findings, evening primrose oil, or gamma linolenic acid, has reduced size of mammary tumors in rats.

GARLIC (Alliatum Satium).

According to many herbal experts, it is a wonder drug of the herbal world. It can act as a natural antibiotic, sometimes called Russian Antibiotic.

Garlic contains vitamins A, B1 and C, and mineral selenium, sulfur, calcium, manganese, copper, iron, potassium, and zinc. Garlic contains the enzymes allinase, peroxidase and myrosinase. It also contains volatile oils composed of allicin; many sulfur related substances, and compounds citral, geranid, linaloal, A-phellendrene, and B-phellendrene. Garlic can be toxic to some tumor cells and is under investigation by the National Cancer Institute for its cancer inhibiting properties. According to research findings, allycin, a compound of garlic, inhibited mammary tumors, and compounds ajoene and diallyl sulfide inhibited liver tumors in rats. According to studies in Italy and China, people who have diets rich in garlic and other allium, including onions, have a substantially lower occurrence of stomach cancer.

CAUTION!!—Garlic shouldn't be used by breast feeding mothers.

Also, eating of 10 or more of garlic cloves a day can cause allergies/be toxic. Do not overdose it!

GINGER ROOT (Zangiber Officinale)

Ginger Root contains vitamin A, B complex, C, and minerals calcium, phosphorus, iron, sodium, potassium, and magnesium. It also contains oil called ginerol. It is believed that this oil acts as a "transporter" of other herbs to the organs they are designed to heal. It also has detoxifying properties; according to research findings, it neutralizes carcinogens produced by charbroiling of meat. Chinese ginger compounds have shown inhibitive action against liver cancer.

GINGKO (Ginkgo Biloba)

Gingko contains flatten glycosides, that have strong antioxidant properties. Gingko stimulates immune system. Gingko improves blood flood to the brain, and protects nerve tissues from degeneration.

GINSENG (Korean: Panax Shin-Seng
        Siberian: Eletherococcus
        Wild American: Panax Quinque Folium)

The main active ingredients in ginseng are called ginsenosides. According to experts, the higher the quantity of ginsenosides, the better the quality of the ginseng. Ginseng contains vitamins B1, B2, B3, B5, biotin, rutin, vitamins A, E, and minerals calcium, iron, phosphorus, sodium, silicon, potassium, manganese, magnesium, sulfur, tin and germanium.

Germanium possibly enables the blood malignant cells to attract oxygen, and become normal, so it may help to inhibit growth of cancerous tumors.

Ginseng is very popular among Chinese herbalists that use it for a variety of ailments. It also has a stimulating effect on the body, and can increase its energy and stamina.

CAUTION!!—do not take ginseng together with vitamin C—wait for two hours after taking vitamin C!

GOLDEN SEAL (Hydrastis Canadensis)

Golden seal is believed to be helpful against stomach, uterus, ovary and lip cancers. Golden seal contains vitamins A, B complex, C, E and F.

It also has minerals calcium, copper, potassium, phosphorus, manganese, iron, zinc and sodium. It contains hydrastine that gives the golden seal its antibiotic, anti-viral properties. It also contains berberine that helps to eliminate growth of harmful bacteria, Candida Albicans, inside the digestive system. It is also an excellent laxative.

Additionally, it has the ability to lower blood sugar level. Diabetics and people with normal sugar can use it.

It shouldn't be used by hypoglycemics (Persons with low sugar level).

GREEN TEA (Camelia Sinensis)

It was found that the green tea can help to prevent stomach cancer, and it can be helpful against other types of cancer.

Polyphenols, the compounds of green tea have antioxidant properties, and can inhibit formation of carcinogens.

FO-TI or HO SHOU WU (Polygonum Multiflorum)

It is a popular herb in China. This herb may prevent cancer; animal tests using Fo-Ti Extracts have shown its antitumor activity.

LICORICE ROOT (Glycyrrhiza Glabra)

Licorice contains vitamin B—complex, pantothenic acid, niacin, biotin, vitamin E, phosphorus, lecithin, manganese, iodine, chromium and zinc.

Licorice also contains glycirrhizinic acid. The Japanese are currently investigating glycyrrhizinic acid as a possible cancer treatment agent. In the United States, the National Cancer Institute investigates triterpenoids, compounds found in the licorice root, for their ability to inhibit growth of cancerous cells/9/.

CAUTION!!—Licorice has high content of sugar, and should be used by diabetics very cautiously. It can also raise blood pressure, so people with high blood pressure shouldn't use it In high quantities, it can also deprive potassium from the body, so the potassium level should be checked once in a while, and potassium be supplemented/7/.

POKE WEED or POKE ROOT (Phytolacca Americana)

Poke root has been used in folk medicine against breast cancer. Poke root makes a good poultice for breast tumors and caked breasts. The poultice should be made by grinding the root into powder, and mixing it with the Slippery Elm herb, and water. Apply it to the swellings and remoisten it when it dries. Keep the poltice on all day, and change it every three days/4/.

PACIFIC YEW (Taxus Brevifolia)

Pacific yew tree is a source of taxol that was found to be effective in about 30 % of patients with advanced ovarian cancer.

PAU D'ARCO (see TAHEEBO)

RED CLOVER (Triforium Pratense)

According to Jehtro Kloss and other herbalists, it is one of nature's best herbs, and excellent blood purifier. Combined with equal parts of blue violet, burdock, yellow dock, dandelion root, rock rose and golden seal it can help in treating cancerous growths/4/.

Red clover is believed to be efficient against cancer in any part of the body. Jehtro Kloss recommended that for throat cancer, one should gargle a strong red clover tea three to four times daily, and then swallow it.

For stomach cancer, four or more cups of red clover tea on an empty stomach should be drunk. For rectum cancer, internal injection, five or six times daily, is recommended.

For uterus cancer, the tea should be injected into vagina, and kept after injection, for several minutes/4/.

Red clover can be especially beneficial against Esophageal and mammary cancers.

Red clover contains vitamins A, B-complex, C, F, and P. It also contains minerals iron, phosphorus, magnesium, calcium, copper, selenium, cobalt, nickel, manganese, sodium, molybdenum and tin.

Red clover is a compound of Harry Hoxsey's anticancer formula.

I believe that a red clover herb is a MUST in each cancer treatment; take this herb on a daily basis (Powdered, in a capsule form, three capsules three times daily.)

REISHI MUSHROOM (Ganoderma Lucidum)

Recent studies show that extract from this Chinese mushroom can stop the growth of cancerous tumors in mice/9/.

SANICLE (Sanicula Marilandica)

It is one of "cure-all-" herbs. It heals both internal and external wounds and tumors.

Drinking of a sanicle tea (1 teaspoon per 1 cup of water, boiled for half an hour), five or six times a day is recommended/4, 9/.

SLIPPERY ELM BARK (Ulmus Vulva)

Slippery elm contains the vitamin C, E, F, K, and P. It also contains minerals iron, sodium, calcium, selenium, iodine, copper, manganese, zinc, potassium, and phosphorus.

It is helpful in reducing inflammation of the mucus membranes of the mouth, throat and lungs and it relieves both constipation and diarrhea. It enhances output of corvine hormone by adrenal glands.

It has been used in a treatment of cancer. Together with burdock, sorrel and Indian turkey rhubarb it is a compound of Hoxsey's and Caisse's formulas.

SHIITAKE MUSHROOM (Lentinus Edoles)

This mushroom contains a polysaccharide called Lentinan that slows growth of cancerous tumors in animals. It is presently used as cancer fighting agent in China and Japan.

SPIRULINA

Spirulina is rich in nutrients. Spirulina is believed to be helpful in cancer prevention therapy; it helps to eliminate radiation poisoning, and it can help to prevent kidneys failure during chemotherapy.

TA—HEEBO INNER BARK or PAU D'ARCO or IPE ROXO

Ta Heebo contains mineral iron and zinc. Research in South America and in the United States show that an extract from the tree bark contains lapachol, with active ingredients effective against some forms of cancer. Ta Heebo/Pau D'Arco is presently used in some hospitals in Brazil in cancer therapy. It is believed to be helpful against pancreatic, prostate, intestinal, lung, brain and other cancers.

It also has antibiotic properties with virus killing ability. It is very useful against parasitic and fungal infections. It lowers blood sugar, so it may help to prevent diabetes.

Ta Heebo Tea is one of the ingredients of Jonathan Winter's Miracle Cancer Cure Tea/9/.

I believe that Taheebo/Pau D'Arco bark is a MUST for cancer patients; drink a Pau D'Arco extract three times daily (Diluted with water, one to two table-spoons, three times daily.)

TURMERIC

The curry spice turmeric, according to study performed in 2002 at Kumamoto University in Japan, could help prevent and possibly cure cancer. Turmeric contains an ingredient called cur cumin that was found to inhibit production of interleukin-8 (IL-8), which is suspected of stimulating cancer cells to produce while at the same time suppressing the immune system. In a study performed at the University of Rochester Medical Center, New York State, USA, it was found that cur cumin helped protect the skin of cancer patients who were undergoing radiation therapy. In addition, the cur cumin was found to suppress the development of new cells in tumors.

WILD YAM (Diocorea Villosa)

When combined with other blood cleaners, it can aid in removing wastes from the system. Wild Yam has steroid-like substances, and is present in many gland balancing formulas, including birth control pills. It contains DHEA that is believed to be helpful against skin, lung, colon, liver, breast and lymphatic cancers.

Wild yam is recommended by some experts as possibly being excellent for gall bladder and liver diseases, and it can counteract nausea (for nausea, use it in a two ounce dosage, with some honey added)/4, 9/.

YELLOW DOCK (Rumex Crispas)

According to research findings, emodin, a compound of yellow dock, is active against cancers lymphocyte leukemia and Walker carcinosarcoma. Yellow dock has also shown beneficial effect against glandular tumors.

HERBAL PREPARATIONS AND USING OF HERBS

Some herbs (leaves and flowers) should be taken in a powdered form only. They should be dried in normal temperatures (freezing and thermal processing should be avoided!)

Other "herb" forms, such as tree bark and roots, must be specially prepared—their properties are only preserved if they are taken in an extract or a tea form.

Recommendations on herbal preparations and using of herbs are shown below;

TEA/DECOCTION/; a tea made of the ROOTS and BARK. Use 1 teaspoon of the powdered or 1 tablespoon of cut herb on a cup of water. Gently boil for 30 minutes. Let stand 10 minutes.

EXTRACT: Extracts are commercially made liquid solvents into which the principal ingredients of HERB POWDERS are soluble. The cold percolation of the herb with a solvent (for example, alcohol, water, grape brandy, or apple cider vinegar), extracts the herb of its nutrients factors, trace minerals and enzymes. Extracts are absorbed in the body much faster and can be used by a person having difficulties in swallowing capsules, small children, etc.

To make an extract, you should soak a proper quantity of herb, in a solvent (I use a Bacardi rum), for at least a two weeks time. Only a glass container must be used!

FOMENTATION; A fomentation is made from a cloth soaked in a hot tea (infusion or Decoction) applied to the effected area. Poultice is more effective than fomentation.

TEA/INFUSION; A tea is made of the LEAVES AND BLOSSOMS.

Use 1 teaspoon of the POWDERED herb. Bring 1 cup of the water to boiling, add the herb, cover and steep for 10 minutes.

OIL OF HERBS: It is an extraction of the herb in an oil base.

Place the POWDERED herb at the top of the double boiler; cover with OLIVE OIL, Cook (on low heat) for 3.5 hours, extract the oil. Store in dark glass bottles.

POULTICE; It is a moist, herbal pack applied locally. Mix the powdered herb with warm water, spread on a clean cloth and cover the effected area.

TINCTURE (same as extract)—It is an extract of herbs in alcohol or vinegar (Alcohol is much better.) Cover four ounces of herb with one pint of alcohol (190 proof or other). Store in a glass jar for 2 weeks; mix or shake 1–2 times daily. Use 1–2 teaspoons of tincture, 3–4 times daily, with water or juice.

If you cannot use the alcohol, you can steep the tincture for a few minutes on a low heat, until the alcohol evaporates, then use it. You can prepare the extract yourself. Tincture is more efficient then tea or capsule in the case when the bark or root of tree/herb is used.

A Basic Review of the Alternative/Holistic Cancer Therapies

1

INHIBITION OF GROWTH
OF NEW BLOOD VESSELS
(ANGIOGENESIS)

According to research findings angiogenesis inhibitors are substances that inhibit development of new blood vessels' network. In this way, both tumor growth and the spread of cancer through metastasis can be inhibited.

CARTILAGE

Of thirteen substances researched by Dr. Folkman, only cartilage didn't show any toxicity. Other substances cannot be used for a prolonged time, because they are toxic. Also, the cartilage has shown highest angiogenesis inhibition rate according to CAM index.

ANGIOSTATIN

The experiments with mice, performed in 1994 at Children's Hospital in Boston, by scientists who included Dr. Judah Folkman, have indicated that large tumors produce a protein, called angiostatin that inhibits the growth of tiny secondary tumors elsewhere in the body.

It was found, that large cancer tumors produce not only large amount of substances that stimulate new blood vessel growth, but they also produce smaller amount of inhibitor, angiostatin. Both stimulators and inhibitors are released into the bloodstream, but while the stimulators disappear quickly; the inhibitors can concentrate in large quantities. When the large tumor is removed, the content of angiostatin goes down, and rapid growth of metastases can occur.

In summary, angiostatin, that can be isolated from enzyme precursor plasminogen, is a natural substance produced by a human body that regulates the formation of new blood vessels. While injected in mice with large tumors, angiostatin has prevented the development of metastases. Further efforts are under way to produce enough material to begin clinical trials in humans.

INHIBITION OF ANGIOGENESIS WITH CARTILAGE

According to research findings by Dr. Folkman, tumor growth is dependent upon the growth of new blood vessels. It means that tumors can not grow and metastasize without the network of blood vessels that nourish them.

If the development of blood vessels is inhibited, the growth of tumors and metastasis is also inhibited—they simply die.

The studies that were performed to find effective angiogenesis inhibitor had found that such an inhibitor can be a cartilage.

Cartilage is avascular/without blood vessels/, and it has an ability of keeping blood vessels of, preventing them from developing on it (blood vessels appear on cartilage only during a fetal stage, or in arthritic condition, leading to calcification of cartilage). According to Patricia D'Amore Ph.D., of the Laboratory of Surgical Research, at the Children Hospital in Boston, the avascular tissue extracts contain inhibitors of angiogenesis/5/.

Research was performed using calves' cartilage to define if it can inhibit the vascularization of solid tumors, at the Massachusetts Institute of Technology. The findings reported by a research team of Dr. Robert Layer Sc.D. and Anna Lee Ph.D., in the Journal "Science", have confirmed that the cartilage found in the shoulders of calves can inhibit vascularization of solid tumors. Later on, these scientists performed similar research using shark cartilage.

Experiments performed by Carl Luer Ph.D., at the Mote Marine Laboratory in Sarasota, Florida, have shown that the sharks exposed to high levels of carcinogenic substances, didn't show any higher incidents of cancer and tumors, opposite to other animals exposed to similar conditions.

Sharks have a strong and very effective immune system. They are largely free of infections. Antibodies contained in the shark blood successfully combat bacteria and viral infections, and provide protection against many chemicals that are life threatening to most mammals.

It was discovered that sharks have a peculiar immunoglobin in their blood that is probably responsible for their immune resistance. Also, testing of protein extracts from the cartilage has shown that there are six or seven proteins that have ability to prevent blood vessels' growth.

Also, complex muccosaccarides in cartilage, probably have immune-regulatory and angiogenesis inhibiting effect.

The cartilage is a substance made mostly from undifferentiated bone cells that become chondrocytes, cartilage cells producing intertuning cartilaginous fibers. It is a tough, elastic, and translucent material. There are three types of cartilage, and strongest one, the fibrocartilage, is found between backbones.

According to William Lane, co-author of the book "Sharks do not get cancer"/5/ the dried shark cartilage has the following properties;

- The main components are ash (about 41%), protein (about 39%) carbohydrates (about 12%), water (about 7%), fiber (less then 1%) and fat (less then 0.3%). The ash consists mostly of calcium and phosphorus; those are necessary nutrients for the body. The muccosaccarides that are in the carbohydrates stimulate a body's immune system. The proteins (macro proteins) appear to carry angiogenesis inhibitors that prevent growth of blood vessels. It is very important that the cartilage be properly prepared; it shouldn't be exposed to heat while dried (raw cartilage contains more then 85% water). The best cartilage should be freeze dried, and finely milled. It was found that shark cartilage is about 1000 more effective then the bovine (calf) cartilage.

It is very important that the protein content of the cartilage be absorbed BEFORE it is digested by enzymes. Once digested, the protein is broken down into aminoacids that are not as effective as angiogenesis inhibitors.

Absorption can be accomplished from the intestine via oral administration, or from any other cavity or part in the body.

The studies performed by Dr. Prudden on 31 patients with variety of cancers and tumors have indicated that **bovine cartilage** has caused complete tumor regression in 35 % of patients, a complete response with relapse was observed in 26 %, and a partial response in 19 %. The research findings of Dr.Prudden's experiments printed in the Journal of Biological Response Modifiers stated, that in case of pancreatic cancer, squamous or adenocarcinoma of the lung, glioblastama multiforme, and similar diseases, where conventional methods are unsuccessful, the use of "Catrix" (powdered calf cartilage) therapy should be considered.

Additionally, calf cartilage therapy, in contrast to chemotherapy, damages no "immunological or hematological bridges"/5/.

The studies performed by Dr. Brian G.M. Durie at the Department of Internal Medicine at the University of Arizona Health Sciences Center **indicated that the bovine cartilage applied directly to cancer tumor cells from fresh biopsy specimens in test tubes killed ovarian, pancreatic, colon, testicular, and sarcoma tumor cells.**

The studies performed by Dr. Contreas on 8 patients with advanced, inoperable, cancers, have indicated that the **shark cartilage** had caused a reduction in tumor size of 30 to 100 percent in 7 of the patients.

In other studies performed by Dr. Elia Ferguson Ph.D. in Panama, have shown a positive response to shark cartilage in patient with terminal pulmonary cancer and in the patient with advanced liver tumor/5/.

RECOMMENDATIONS

According to some experts both bovine and shark cartilage has shown beneficial results against heavily vascularized SOLID TUMORS, such as BREAST, CERVICAL, PROSTATE, CENTRAL NERVOUS SYSTEM, BRAIN, PANCREATIC and similar cancers. Recently, the bovine cartilage is recommended as showing much better results against vascularized tumor growth.

Cancers such as lymphoma, Hodgkin's, and leukemia are less likely to respond to treatment with cartilage.

According to the literature review/5/, approximately 1.2 gram per each 2.2 pounds (1-kilogram) of body weight is suggested to limit the tumor growth in advanced stages (stage 3 and 4) of cancer development.

Usually, approximately 60 grams of cartilage on a daily basis, for normal weight person is recommended.

These 60 grams of conventional cartilage (with protein content between 38 and 43 percent, freeze dried), may be taken orally (in four, 15 grams doses, mixed with vegetable juice; carrot, beet or tomato), preferably about 15 minutes before meals, first time in the morning, last time during the day at the bedtime.

If you have a digestive system problem, the cartilage may be administered rectally (also this assures better absorption). As a retention enema, mix 15 grams of cartilage powder with two-thirds to one cup of water at a body temperature.

Preliminary results/5/indicate that some reduction in tumor size may be noted within 6 weeks after the treatment and major tumor reduction may be noted within 11 weeks. When tumors are less life threatening, this dosage can be reduced up to 60 percent.

As a preventive measure, about 7 to 8 grams of cartilage (9–12 tablets) daily may help to prevent reoccurrence, for a person with normal body weight.

CAUTION!!!—Cartilage is not recommended for pregnant women (they have to build blood network for developing fetus), and for people who recently had deep surgery and need new blood vessels. It is also not advised for people who recently suffered a heart attack, as well as for people in a major muscle building program.

2

REVIEW OF OTHER HOLISTIC CANCER THERAPIES

According to Drs.K.W.Donsbach, D.C., N.D., Ph.D., H.R. Asleben, M.D., D.O., Ph.D., authors of the "Holistic Cancer Therapy"/2/, there are several alternative cancer treatments that are popular worldwide, however, they are not practiced yet in the United States, the main reason being long and expensive drug approval procedure by FDA.

A very short review and description of alternative cancer treatments, with emphasizes on the particular cancers are included for your information. However, I advise that you should seek an advice of a reputable nutritionist/doctor practicing a natural healing in you area, before undertaking any of these treatments on your own.

According to Drs. Donsbach and Asleben, they have got very good results with inoperable, terminally ill cancer patients, at the hospitals they operate in Mexico and Poland; Hospital Santa Monica, Hospital St. Augustine, and Institute Santa Monica.

WARNING: there are many international clinics offering alternative cancer therapies you can find more information about them in the "Third Opinion; An International Directory to Alternative Therapy Centers for the Treatment and Prevention of Cancer" by John Fink/21/), however, before you commit yourself to any of them, first ask for their percentage of recovery, and if possible, try to contact personally and see the people who have recovered there. Many of these clinics may act under false pretences!

Below is short overview of holistic therapies:

PULSE MODULATED MICROWAVE HYPOTHERMIA

According to Dr. Donsbach/2/this therapy may possibly introduce damage to cancer cells without damaging normal tissue.

The Pulse—Modulated Microwave Hypothermia may be used to treat cancer anywhere in the body/2/. Rectal—colon, vaginal, breast, and lung cancers as well as skin, liver, vagina, brain tumors and enlarged prostate glands can be treated by employing this method.

- THYMUS THERAPY AND THYMUS GLAND RESTORATION

Thymus activation therapy, originally developed in Sweden more than 40 years ago, is essential in cancer treatment. Thymus gland is responsible for proper functioning of the immune system.

Proper nutrition and concentrated nutrients such as pantothenic acid and vitamin A May enhance thymus gland function/2, 7/.

The thymus gland supplements, Bee Propolis and Echinacea herb may be beneficial in thymus gland strengthening.

- HYDRAZINE SULFATE

The developing cancer cell needs energy from the glucose. Lactic acid is a by-product of the breakdown of the glucose in cancer cell. Lactic acid is converted into glucose again by the kidneys and the liver. According to Dr. Donsbach/2/a substance hydrazine sulfate may inhibit the production of glucose from lactic acid in the liver; with this safe and effective means of controlling the spread of cancer, the regression of tumor masses may be achieved.

- HIGH pH THERAPY WITH CESIUM CHLORIDE

Since all cancer cells are acid due to presence of lactic acid in them, the reduction of their acidity through increasing pH inside these cells can slow their growth.

According to Drs. Donsbach and Alsleben/2/, when cesium is applied to cancer patients, it enters the cancer cells and makes their interior alkaline. It was found that pH of cancer cells equal to 7.6 stops the growth of cancer, and at pH 8 to 8.5, the life of cancer cells is limited to only several hours.

According to the pioneer in high pH-therapy, Dr. Keith Brewer, this method is not toxic to normal cells, opposite to other methods producing cells' alkalinity.

This method may be effective in the following treatments;

- Suppression and regression of SARCOMA

- BRONCHOGENIC CARCINOMA with bone metastasis

- COLON CANCER

Also studies show that this method can be effective against other cancers/2/.

LAETRILE (AMYGDALIN, VITAMIN B-17)

This method was developed by Ernst Krebs, Jr.Ph.D. who applied the John's Beard's theory that cancer cells grow from the displaced trophoblast cells, e.g. cells existing in human uterus during first weeks of pregnancy.

Most of these cells are killed by a pancreatic enzyme Chymotrypsin. Since Laetrile can act in similar way as Chymotrypsin, it possibly may also be used to kill growing cancer cells.

Laetrile is found in over 1,200 different plants, including seeds of such common fruits as apricots, apples, peaches and plums. It may be taken as a preventive measure, or as a metabolic treatment against cancer. It shouldn't be overdosed—it can be toxic in bigger quantities. According to Jason Winters, one 500 mg. Laetrile tablet should be taken thirty minutes before each meal, after three pancreatic enzymes.

According to Drs. Donsbach and Alsleben/2/there are other, better methods then this one. A one study performed at the Mexican clinic, on the seventeen patients treated with the laetrile tablets indicated that none of the patients survived more than 3 years.

So be very careful/seek a second opinion before taking this supplement.

- GERMANIUM

Since anaerobic cancer cells can't live in high-oxygen environment, the use of substance enhancing oxygen can help in curing cancer.

Germanium may act as an oxygen enhancer, and it possibly also stimulates the body's own natural defense system. The plants rich in germanium are shiitake mushrooms, ginseng, and garlic.

- DIMETHYL SULFOXIDE (DMSO)

The research performed at Mt. Sinai Hospital has shown that when DMSO was injected into leukemic mice, the leukemic cancer cells began to perform as normal cells/2/.

In LEUKEMIA CANCER, the body is saturated with immature white cells that do not mature. DMSO probably causes that these immature cells "grow up" and become functional.

DMSO also can possibly assist many other cancer treating substances, and can be also beneficial in many other diseases. Additionally, it doesn't have any harmful side effects (However, this food supplement shouldn't be taken together with the conventional medications, and shouldn't be mixed or taken at the same time with other food supplements.)

- CHLODRONATE

According to Drs. Donsbach and Alsleben/2/this substance may be especially beneficial to BONE CANCER patients.

The bone cancer is a result of metastasis of breast or prostate cancer. Chlodronate may reduce pain and may prevent the bone cancer from further spreading.

There is no sufficient evidence that Chlodronate actually cures bone cancer, and it is hardly, in only 2% absorbed by the body. It is not approved by FDA.

According to the recent research, zoledronate (Zometa) supplements (4 to 8 Mg) have shown much better results in preventing metastasis of cancer to the bones. Zometa is FDA approved.

- LHRH AND FLUTAMIDE THERAPIES (LABRIE PROTOCOL)

The Leutinizing Hormone—releasing-Hormone (LRHH) and Flutamide therapy can be especially beneficial against PROSTATE CANCER, under condition those patients were previously not treated with estrogen/2, 16/.

Dr. F. Labrie of Quebec University, Quebec, Canada, developed this method. He has found that a "Lupron Depot" drug, applied together with Flutamide will lower androgen hormones in males.

According to Drs. Donsbach and Alsleben/2/within 5 days of initiating the above therapy in prostate cancer patients, the level of prostatic acid phosphatase ("marker" used to check the progress of prostate cancer), started to decrease in these patients by about 50%, and in two months time, 90% of these patients were cured and had a normal level of prostatic acid phosphatase.

Even advanced cases of prostate cancer, with metastasis to bones, can be cured with this method. In patients previously treated with estrogen, the LHRH and Flutamide therapy is no longer beneficial, since the cancer will not react to these substances; however, other alternative treatment methods may be successful.

- LIVE CELL THERAPY

In this treatment, the extracted DNA of liver, pancreas, thymus, adrenal, spleen etc. glands are injected as natural stimulant to the patient's own DNA.

The use of extracted DNA from animal organs began many years ago—unborn animals' organs were used because these extracts do not cause an immune defense reaction. Though Live Cell Therapy will not work on cancer cells directly, it can help to energize a starved and tired of a long illness body.

- CARBATINE

This therapy is based on the healing effect of urine in certain conditions. It was shown both in laboratory and clinical studies that the urea is effective against variety of malignancies.

The substance carbatine contains urea and creatine hydrate, both of which have been reported to have anti-cancer properties. The ingredients of carbatine have the ability to interfere with metabolic exchanges and replication processes leading to uncontrolled growth of cancer cells.

LIVER AND BONE CANCER may react to the addition of carbatine to the treatments/2/.

- ONCOTOX

Oncotox contains an Ortho-Para-Toluene-Sul-Fonamide compound CgH13O2NS. It was shown at the Mallory Institute of Pathology, Boston School of Medicine, which the Oncotox can enhance both B and T cells response to Mitigen and can enhance Natural Killer Cells activity. According to research studies, Oncotox may inhibit tumor growth and mitosis in only four days. Though it can kill cancer cells, and may inhibit their reproduction, it doesn't have any such effect on normal cells/2/.

- HYDROGEN PEROXIDE

The experiment of infusing hydrogen peroxide prior to the radiation therapy and later to the use of chemotherapy was performed at Totton University School of Medicine, Japan. Patients with MAXILLARY CANCER showed a promising response to this infusion; 8 patients out of 15 have shown almost complete disappearance of the tumor, 6 have shown partial reduction, and only one had a small change.

However, this method can have **severe adverse** side effects, and if improperly applied, can **be very dangerous. A patient can not employ it** himself—it can be employed only by very experienced medical staff, if at all…Since it is very easy to overdose this substance, any misuse of hydrogen peroxide can cause additional pain and destruction of blood!

One MUST be very careful with this treatment—always seek a second opinion!

- COENZYME COQ-10

According to Drs. Donsbach and Alsleben/2/this substance is used mostly as an addition to Anti-cancer drug Adriamycin. Adriamycin depletes COQ-10 in the heart muscle, so when COQ-10 is administered together with this drug, the damage can be prevented.

Though COQ-10 probably doesn't have anti-cancer activity itself, it enhances other body's functions, thus controlling cancer development.

- IMMUNE—MODULATION THERAPY

Drs. Donsbach and Alsleben/2/recommend this therapy as implementation of miscellaneous vaccines that aid the body against various harmful biological agents, including Kleptic TM microbes and other agents that can cause cancer and other diseases. Seek a second opinion about this treatment!

- IMMUNE-AUGMENTATIVE THERAPY

Immune-Augmentative Therapy (IAT), developed by Dr. L. Burton, involves injections of vaccines of processed blood products that contain cancer-inhibiting components. Up to four components, of the immune system, extracted from the blood can be employed in this experimental treatment.

Three of these components consist of 2 tumor antibodies and a deblocking protein. The fourth factor, called tumor complement TC, is derived from the blood clots of cancer patients. The information about this therapy may be available available at Dr. Lawrence Burrton's Immunology Research Center (IRC) on Grand Bahamas Island/2/.

- ANTINEOPLASTONS

The antineoplastons are natural components that are produced by human body. These components are present in a blood and urine of healthy people, but they are low or absent in cancer affected people.

These components were discovered by Dr. Stanislaw Burzynski of Burzynski Research Institute in Houston, Texas, as having anti-tumor activity. According to research findings, antineoplastons are components of a biochemical defense system that works parallel to the immune system.

While the immune system defends body through destruction of external invaders or defective cells, the biochemical defense system is responsible for regulation and normalization of the defective cells, including cancerous cells. Antineoplastons are chemical substances, part of compounds called peptides, from the blood protein family; those are responsible for transmitting the information to the cells.

Four antineoplastons named A2, A5, A10, and AS2-1 are used by Dr. Burzynski, in cancer patients' treatment.

According to his research findings, these non-toxic antineoplastons have shown a considerable shrinkage of tumors in cases where conventional medicine couldn't help. According to these findings, more than 60 % of the patients treated at the Burzynski Research Institute showed considerable improvement during phase 1 testing/16/.

3

IN SEARCH OF MISSING GENES

Several scientists, frustrated by inefficiency and side effects of traditional cancer treatments such as radiation and chemotherapy, have started research on cancer on a molecular level.

The studies involved studies of tumor cells DNA and the oncogenes (genes that stimulate the uncontrolled cell division), and tumor suppression genes (genes that prevent cells from dividing).

One of the research teams, led by Robert Weiberg at the Whitehead Institute for Biomedical Research in Cambridge, Massachusetts, has, as one of the first, positively identified, isolated and sequenced an oncogene in mammals/8/. They have researched an oncogene called Her-2/neu. They have found that this oncogene's protein product worked as a surface receptor. This receptor is sitting on a surface of the cell and acts in antenna-like manner, receiving signals from the environment. These signals are telling the cells to divide and reproduce continuously.

The knowledge of this oncogene protein product, its location, and activities has helped to develop therapies that can target this particular protein.

Further studies were performed where the human version of oncogene Her-2/neu protein was injected into mice. In response, the mice have produced an antibody that recognize and attacks the human tumor protein cell.

The research team in collaboration with a biotechnology company Genotech has isolated the genes that direct the production of these antibodies. These genes were injected into the culture of mouse cells that in response have produced the antibodies.

The experiments have shown that these antibodies have stopped the growth of human tumors transplanted into mice. Further experimental studies on using these antibodies on women with breast cancer have shown very promising results.

More advanced version of the antibodies is now being elaborated at Genetech, consisting of a stretch of mouse DNA and a piece of human antibody gene/8/.

However, the oncogene Her-2/neu, responsible mostly for breast cancers, is only one between many other oncogenes, responsible for other types of cancer. There are many different genes mutations that can cause uncontrolled cell division in other kinds of cancer. To find these other genes, it is necessary to look into almost 3 billion base pairs of DNA stretch 100,000 genes, and 23 chromosomes.

In heditary cancer diseases, gene hunting is a laborious and repetitive process—the inheritance pattern is searched in segments of chromosomes of family members that could have inherited the disease, and then, by a comparison, a "faulty" gene can be identified. Once this gene is found, a person can undergo regular check-ups and a preventive surgery can be performed at the beginning of cancer development, before cancer grows and metastasizes further.

This method is being used, for example, in the treatment of an eye cancer retinoblastoma. Since the gene causing this cancer has been identified, the patients at the risk of developing this kind of cancer (mostly children, carrying this inherited gene), can undergo regular check-ups, and the tumors can be destroyed by a safe laser surgery just at the beginning of their growth. Further research about the oncogenes and their protein products will lead to new preventive and curative therapies.

But maybe, one day, it will be also discovered that some herbal and other natural therapies contain the elements that have the oncogene regulating properties?

4

NEVER, NEVER GIVE UP!

I would like to finish this guide with a story, which I believe is very interesting—a real life happening that was described by Jethro Kloss, a distinguished pioneer on herbal therapy in his fundamental book "Back to Eden"/4/.

This story describes a treatment that was performed on one of his patients, a woman with a cancer that has spread all over her body, including her entire abdomen.

Her surgeon has found her inoperable and sent her home, saying that she would live "no more than 3 to 10 days". The only medication given to her was pain relievers.

When she was seen by J. Kloss, nothing could pass through her bowels, and waste matter and urine was coming through surgically made openings.

At the beginning of her treatment by J. Kloss, she was given herbal enemas that cleaned her bowels, so she started to have bowel movements through her rectum, and she could start taking herbal teas and fruit juice.

After the artificially made openings healed, she was able to start taking warm baths. She was given warm, sweat baths every day, followed by salt glows, cold towel rubs, and massage. She also had fomentation every day over her entire abdomen area (liver, stomach, spleen, spine), after which her entire back and abdomen were saturated with herbal liniment.

This liniment consisted of 2 ounces of powdered myrrh, one ounce of powdered golden seal, one-half ounce of cayenne pepper, and 1 quarter of 70% rubbing alcohol that were mixed together, shaken every day while bottled in glass container, for 7 days.

Additionally, her entire abdomen was massaged several times a day.

She also enjoyed sunshine, fresh air and rest.

During this time, she took all advised by Mr. Kloss herbs, and was on a proper diet, eating plenty of leafy green vegetables, and fresh, vine-ripened tomatoes. This treatment was followed for about four months, until her condition has improved.

Since then, she enjoyed a long, cancer-free, healthy life.

This story is a best summary of natural cancer therapy that can be recommended to anybody.

However, on the basis of my review, I would like to repeat again the most important items of a natural cancer therapy. Also, it is desirable that you search for and read some of the books on your own, since many of them contain rich, real life experiences of cancer survivors and/or important research findings and you can benefit more if you personally become familiar with the available literature.

SUMMARY OF THE CANCER PREVENTION AND HEALING THERAPY

The most important is to keep your blood and your lymphatic system clean from toxins, so there will be no support in your blood to a growth of fungi, viruses, cancer and other diseases.

The properly nourished and oxygenated body will better resist and fight foreign "invaders" including cancer growth.

You—through your mind power should help your body to fight your enemy—cancer.

The natural cancer prevention/healing therapy should be started with a proper **cleansing/purifying diet** consisting mainly of fruit juices (made of one fruit—do not mix any fruits together) and herbal teas, alternatively taken, every 1 hour (See chapter on fruits for the fruit selection.)

This fasting diet should be followed for 3 to 10 days, and under the supervision of your nutritionist. At the end of this fasting diet, you may start eating fresh vegetables and fruits, at least four cups daily. Always eat fruit by itself—do not eat it at the same meal with the vegetables, proteins or starches.

However, you can eat vegetables and proteins, and vegetables and starches together.

During this diet, do not eat any meats, diary products, and other "heavy" food. During this fasting diet, to facilitate cleansing of the body from toxins' build-up, you may administer **herbal or black coffee enemas**—for example, an enema made out of three cups of warm coffee, one enema each day.

There are many herbs and herbal compositions that are believed to have beneficial effect against cancer, and they are described in this review—see chapter on herbs.

However, on the basis of many herbal experts' recommendations, the most effective, "main" herbs **are Pau D'Arco (Taheebo) and Red Clover**. You can supplement these main herbs with other herbs, as indicated in this review.

The doses indicated in this review are believed to be helpful as a preventive treatment against cancer.

Caution!—The above therapy should be started **after** a conventional cancer therapy such as surgery and chemotherapy was already completed.

The doses as recommended below should be increased if the cancer was unsuccessfully treated by conventional methods in the past.

- **Pau D'Arco (Ta Heebo)**—since it is a tree bark, for best results use it in a form of an extract/tincture, 1 to 2 tablespoons, three times daily, diluted with water, or herbal teas. Eventually prepare it as a tea.

For a proper preparation/usage, see chapter on herbal preparations.

- **Red clover**—this herb should be taken in a powdered form, in capsules, 3–4 capsules, three times daily.

- Additionally, you may drink herbal teas, for example, Red Clover Formula tea, Jason Winters Tea, etc. Also you may try other blood purifying/system cleansing teas as presented in this review.

Drink herbal teas alternatively with fruit juices—do not mix them or drink them at the same time.

- Drink 2 to 3 cups of freshly squeezed **beet juice**. Also, chlorophyll juices, for example wheat grass juice (best if freshly squeezed), are believed to be beneficial against cancer. Drinking up to four ounces of the wheat grass juice glasses, up to four times daily, is recommended by several herbalists.

- If you can not get these juices freshly squeezed, the brands available in the health stores such as for example a blend of young barley leaves, wheat grass, kelp, brown rice and Bulgarian chlorella, may substitute a fresh juice.

Try to switch to **vegetarian diet**—eat cancer preventive foods that include plenty of raw vegetables, seeds, full grain flour, full grain rye/yeast bread, brown rice, lentils, etc. The proper diet should be rich in fiber, and be from the **alkaline food family**.

However, if you prefer to eat meat, you can consume fish and lean meats (Only in a broiled or cooked form.)

You should avoid the following foods:

- Avoid refined, processed foods, white breads, refined, processed, smoked meats, etc.

- Avoid charred and burned foods.

- No refined (cane, beet, etc.) sugar is allowed. Avoid sweets, cookies, ice cream, sodas, etc. Limit or avoid drinking alcohol (if, only in moderation) and especially, avoid drinking beer.

- Avoid/limit drinking coffee! It may increase "acidity" of your body systems—and cancer thrives when your blood's pH is on an "acid" side!

- Avoid consumption of fat meats, margarine, spreads, etc. You can substitute them with the virgin natural cold pressed olive oil, or canola in moderate quantities, as a fat source—however, a consumption of heated and reheated fats and oils should be totally avoided.

- **Supplements of "antioxidants"** especially such as vitamin A/beta-carotene (precursor of vitamin A), vitamin E, C, zinc and selenium, and supplements of other vitamins and minerals (Potassium) are highly recommended (See chapter on antioxidants and nutrients for recommended quantities.)

- **The thymus gland therapy, as described in this review, may strengthen your immune system**—it includes the thymus gland, echinacea herb, bee propolis and other supplements as further described in this guide.

- **Do not prepare herbs or food in aluminum utensils. Use only stainless steel, glass or ceramic cookware.**

- **Try to avoid taking herbs, when taking medication.** These two usually do not work together.

- If you have a type of cancer that is characterized by a high vascularization (abundant blood network), such as pancreatic, liver, lung and similar cancers, you may supplement your therapy with **a bovine cartilage** in the doses as recommended in this review, together with herbal therapy.

- You may wish to contact some alternative therapy centers for information on treatment offered in their natural healing hospitals. **However, there is a very important warning!!**

Caution!—Before you commit yourself to any of them, first ask for their percentage of recovery, and try to get references and addresses of patients treated there and if possible, contact them personally. You may also want to contact independent nutrition doctors specializing in a natural healing for their opinion about these clinics.

- **Panic is your worst and real enemy.** Positive attitude and positive thinking will help you more in fighting cancer than panic and chaos.

Instead of panicking—meditate and pray.

Look at your life as a beautiful miracle. Think about yourself as an integral part of the Universe. Think about the "creation force"—the Divine Intelligence, God, that has created the Universe and also, has created you. Do not fear Him; do not fear His force, but try to be in harmony with it. Try to love it.

Ask God for help. Trust that you will be helped.

You should be thankful for His help before even you receive it. You must believe that you will be helped.

- Try to live in harmony with yourself and with your environment. Discharge all negative energy, and never get under influence of negative people. See goodness everywhere around you. Love others and love yourself.

Through love, forgiveness and humbleness you will find yourself and the purpose for your life. You will be found by others and loved. You will understand and learn the most important lessons about yourself and about your life.

- Use cancer fighting visualization techniques—listen to the audio-tapes, etc.

- Exercise lightly, enjoy fresh air & outdoors.

- See your doctors regularly, and take prescribed by them treatments and medications.

- The key to good health is taking personal responsibility for it.—<u>Never, never give up</u>!

REFERENCES

1. Cousin, Norman "Head First; the Biology of Hope", 1990, Thorndike Press, Thorndike, Maine

2. Donsbach, Kurt W., Alsleben H. Rudolph, "Holistic Cancer Therapy", 1992, printed in USA, ISBN 0-0963789-24-7.

3. De Camp, Harry S. "Special Report—Mind/Body Power", 1988, Boardroom Reports, Inc. 330 W, 42 St., New York, NY 10036

4. Kloss, Jethro, "Back to Eden—the Classic Guide to Herbal Medicine, Natural Foods, and Home Remedies", 1992, Back to Eden Books Publishing Co., Loma Linda, California 92354

5. Lane, T. William, Comac, Linda "Sharks Do Not Get Cancer—How Shark Cartilage Could Save Your Life", 1992, Avery Publishing Group Inc., Garden City Park, New York

6. Lee, William "Herbs and Herbal Medicine—Their Variety of Uses as Food and Medicine", 1982, Keats Publishing, Inc., Box 876, New Canaan, CT 06840

7. Lepore, Donald, "The Ultimate Healing System. Breakthrough in Nutrition, Kinesiology, and Holistic Healing Techniques" Course Manual, 1988, Woodlands Books, P.O. Box 1422, Provo, Utah 84603

8. Levine, Joseph & Suzuki, David "The Secret of Life—Redesigning the Living World", WGBH Boston, 1993

9. Mindell's Earl "Herb Bible", 1992, Simon & Schuster/Fireside, Simon & Schuster Building, Rockefeller Center, 1230 Avenue of Americas, New York, New York 10020

10. O'Brien, James, "Foods That Fight Breast Cancer", 1993, Globe Communications Corp., 5401 NW Broken Sound Blvd. Boca Raton, FL 33487

11. Royal, Penny C., "Herbally Yours", 1993, Sound Nutrition, P.O.Box 55, Hurricane, Utah 84737

12. Santillo, Humbardt "Natural Healing with Herbs", 1993, Hohm Press, P.O. Box 2501, Prescott, Arizona 86302

13. Siegel, Bernie S., "Peace, Love and Healing. Bodymind Communication and the Path to Self Healing: An Exploration."1989, Harper & Row Publishers, New York

14. "The Healing Foods Cookbook" 400 Delicious Recipes With Curative Power, by the editors of PREVENTION magazine, compiled and edited by Jean Rogers, 1991, Rodale Press, Emmaus, Pennsylvania

15. The Visual Encyclopedia of Natural Healing", A Step-by-Step Pictorial Guide to Solving 100 Everyday Health Problems, by editors of PREVENTION magazine, Health Books, Edited by Alice Feinstein, Rodale Press, Emmaus, Pennsylvania

16. "Cancer Prevention and Nutritional Therapies", by Richard A. Passwater, Ph.D., Keats Publishing, New Canaan, Connecticut

17. Zukav, Gary "The Seat of The Soul", a Fireside Book, published by Simon & Schuster, 1990

18. Winters, Jason; The Jason Winters story by Benjamin Roth Smythe "Killing Cancer" 1980, Vinton Publishing of Las Vegas, 4055 South Spencer Street, Suite 235, Las Vegas, Nevada 89109

19. Anne E. Frahm with David J. Frahm—Cancer Battle Plan—Six Strategies for Beating Cancer from a Recovered "Hopeless Case", 1992, Pinon, PO Box 35007, Colorado Springs, CO 80935

20. Max Gerson, M.D., "A Cancer Therapy, Results of Fifty Cases and the Cure of Advanced Cancer by Diet Therapy"—A Summary of 30 Years of Clinical Experimentation, 1990, Published by The Gerson Institute, PO Box 430, Bonita, CA 91908, in Association with Station Hill Press, Inc. (under The P.U.L.S.E. imprint), Barrytown, New York 12507

21. Fink, John M. "Third Opinion; an International Directory to Alternative Therapy Centers for the Treatment and Prevention of Cancer", 1988, Published by Avery Publishing Inc., Wayne, New Jersey

22. Sommers, Cynthia "Proof Herbs against Cancer", 1994, Red Wing Publishing House, PO BOX 867, Conifer, CO 80433

23. Walters, Richard "Options: The Alternative Cancer Therapy Book", 1993, Avery Publishing Group Inc., Garden City Park, New York

978-0-595-38705-2
0-595-38705-5

www.ingramcontent.com/pod-product-compliance
Lightning Source LLC
Chambersburg PA
CBHW030341290526
45785CB00004B/1559